To Malcol,
vish, Bill

Bill Luckin is Professor of History at the University of Bolton, UK, and former co-editor of *Social History of Medicine*.

DEATH AND SURVIVAL IN URBAN BRITAIN

Disease, Pollution and Environment,
1800–1950

BILL LUCKIN

I.B. TAURIS

LONDON · NEW YORK

Published in hardback in 2015 by
I.B.Tauris & Co Ltd
London • New York
www.ibtauris.com

International Library of Historical Studies 96

ISBN: 978 1 78076 866 3
eISBN: 978 0 85773 977 3

A full CIP record for this book is available from the British Library
A full CIP record is available from the Library of Congress

Library of Congress Catalog Card Number: available

Typeset in Garamond Three by OKS Prepress Services, Chennai, India
Printed and bound by CPI Group (UK) Ltd, Croydon, CR0 4YY

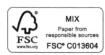

For Carol and David

CONTENTS

FIGURES AND TABLES

PREFACE

This book tells an intellectual, academic and personal story. It charts successive waves of theoretical and methodological change in the linked fields of urban, socio-medical, epidemiological and environmental history. The book also tells a chronological story, or series of linked and layered stories. These revolve around changing patterns of epidemic and endemic disease in British towns and cities between the beginning of the nineteenth century and 1950: the 'discovery' and varying though never less than disturbing impacts of pollution on the quality of urban life during this period: and a predominantly elitist determination to find an 'escape' – a revived and rejuvenated rural alternative – to urban-industrialism. The second part of the book places as much emphasis on the countryside as the city: the one interacted with and partly defined the other. This is the key message of Part 2 of this book.

The first part – 'Disease in the City' – is concerned with cholera, fever and the 'everyday' (but frequently deadly) infections that afflicted the lives of the inhabitants of the capital and the 'new manufacturing districts' between the 1830s and the end of the nineteenth century. A second part – 'Pollution and the Burdens of Urban-Industrialism' – concentrates on the water and 'smoke' problems and the ways in which they (and particularly the latter) came to be perceived, defined and finally brought under a degree of control. A lengthy opening chapter links each of the major themes and sets them in the context of the avalanche of books and journals that has poured from the presses since each of these chapters originally saw the light of day.

An extended conclusion locates the layered and interacting narratives within the framework of the urban revolution that transformed British society between 1800 and 1950. No changes – other than correction of misprints and footnote slips – have been made to previously published material. Retrospective revision would have undermined a major aim: to provide a snap-shot of the state of the art at varying historiographical moments. In this respect, I like to think (though I may be wrong) that the over-simplified and under-documented conclusions to the opening methodological chapter on 'Death and Survival in the City' point as much to the under-developed state of the art in the 1970s as to my own historical immaturity.

Within the disciplinary mainstream, the years between the 1970s and the early twenty first century witnessed a succession of dramatic ideological, conceptual and methodological shifts and debates. The 1970s saw the birth – or was it the reinvention? – of social history. By the end of that decade once highly influential Marxist modes of analysis had entered an era of terminal decline. The void was filled by intense debate – more intense on American campuses than British universities – over structuralism, post-structuralism and the linguistic and cultural turns. In the early 1970s it was possible for a young historian to have a working knowledge of new developments in nearly every area of social history. This is no longer the case. Governments and universities have turned against the social sciences, the arts and humanities. (This, for me, has been the saddest development of the last 40 years.) However, and paradoxically, 'productivity' has increased at an ever more rapid rate. Young historians and established scholars only gain access to scarce research funds if they publish books and journals at a pace that would have astonished my teachers at the London School of Economics in the early 1970s.

There have been other radical changes. In the late 1980s sceptics argued that the 'word' would not survive the stunning impact of new electronic media. This was mistaken. Words are integral to what the internet is and what it does. New electronic media have provided a highly effective vehicle for the delivery of hard-copy journals, original online research and publishing ventures seeking to establish a niche in an ever larger and more diversified range of historical sub-markets. In the future, the internet will become more powerful. Productivity will increase. No historian will be able to read enough, fast enough, to have more than a detailed knowledge of his or her area of expertise and its near neighbours. This is a saddening prospect.

A book like this needs an extra chapter to cover acknowl-edgements. I begin with families. David, Steven, Miles, Joss and Joe Luckin have kept me involved in the joys and problems – far more joys than problems – of being young in the late twentieth and early twenty first centuries. While I was working on the chapters concerned with pollution in the second part of this book, my eldest son David and I met regularly to drink and catch up in south Manchester. This offered me an opportunity periodically to draw on his doctoral expertise in environmental politics, when I was a relative newcomer to that field. More recently, Joss has worked hard on the bibliography when the deadline approached. Quite a long time ago now, Anna, Matthew and Catherine Booth welcomed me to their (and my new) home: Catherine took time out from her sociology degree to retype early journals lost or locked away in the electronic no-person's land of WordPerfect.

Profound thanks to my friends, past and present, at the University of Sussex, the University of Bolton, the Centre for the History of Science, Technology and Medicine at the University of Manchester, the Urban History Group and the Society for the Social History of Medicine. In the late 1990s Graham Mooney and Andrea Tanner made the 'Mortality in the Metropolis' project at the Centre for Metropolitan History at the University of London an intensely enjoyable experience. Graham has continued to keep me up to speed with new developments in socio-medical and demographic history. For a long time now, Joel Tarr at Carnegie-Mellon, Pittsburgh has been inspiration, host and friend. The numerous references to his work show just how much I owe and have learnt from my friend Chris Hamlin, pioneer historian of nineteenth century environmental thought.

In the late 1960s, I worked as secretary for Joseph Needham as he laboured on his super-magnum opus – the multi-volume *Science and Civilisation in China*. During a difficult period in my life he encouraged me to think that it might one day be possible to convert myself into a historian. Nothing would have come of that ambition without the advice and support of Frank Margison who helped me in ways that only he (far more than I) understands. For more than 40 years, Penny Eyles has been a treasured friend. Among much else, our intensely enjoyable conversations have made it possible to escape the obsessively specialized world of historical research. Finally, I want to convey my heartfelt affection for three very special people: Rosalind Williams, Roger Cooter and the late David Sheen. Knowing them has confirmed that I made the right decision when, in the early 1970s, I decided to give up journalism and venture into the world of history. The dedication speaks for itself.

ACKNOWLEDGEMENTS

The previously published chapters in this book first appeared in the following books and journals and are printed by kind permission of the original publishers:

1. *Urban History Yearbook*, 7, 1980, 53–62 (Cambridge University Press).

2. R. Woods and J. Woodward (eds), *Urban Disease and Mortality in Nineteenth Century England* (London: Batsford, 1984).

3. 'The Final Catastrophe: Cholera in London 1866', *Medical History*, 21, 1977, 32–42 (Cambridge University Press).

4. R. Colls and R. Richard (eds), *Cities of Ideas: Civil Society and Urban Governance in Britain 1800–2000: Essays in Honour of David Reeder* (Aldershot: Ashgate, 2004), 46–66.

5. Martin Daunton (ed.), *The Cambridge Urban History of Britain: Volume 3: 1840–1950* (Cambridge: Cambridge University Press, 2000), 207–28.

6. *Social History*, 28, 2003, 31–48 (Taylor and Francis).

7. F. Bosbach, Jens Ivo Engels and Fiona Watson (eds), *Environment and History in Britain and Germany* (Munich: K.G. Saur. Prince Albert Studies Volume 24, 2006), 77–90.

8. Dieter Schott, Bill Luckin and Genevieve Massard-Guilbaud (eds), *Resources of the City: Contributions to an Environmental History of Modern Europe* (Aldershot: Ashgate, 2005), 230–45.

PART 1

DISEASE IN THE CITY

CHAPTER 1

COUNTRY, TOWN AND 'PLANET' IN BRITAIN 1800-1950

An unknown historical territory

Venturing uncertainly into the history of environment and disease in the early 1970s proved an anxiety-inducing experience. Monographs were rare, specialist journals even rarer.[1] To the uninitiated, medical history seemed to offer a promising point of entry. Not so. With a handful of exceptions, scholars in the field were committed to exploring what would soon come to be known as 'internal' issues.[2] Little had been written about the grassroots historical experience of urban (or rural) death, survival and environmental deprivation. Victims of disease were barely visible.[3]

The early 1970s saw the emergence of a new social history of medicine. The sub-discipline focused on relationships between the medical and epidemiological past and the larger society in which they were then believed to be non-problematically located. The new field prospered. Over the next 40 years it expanded and diversified, spawning specialist journals, an international research community and hundreds of conferences.[4] From the 1990s onwards, a minority of writers, influenced by the cultural turn, began to question the utility of the 'social' as an explanatory category, and to interrogate the value of a now widely used term – 'context' – in which everything medical was claimed to have been situated.[5] But theoretical and methodological critique made little impact on the way in which most social historians of medicine went about their business, although theory – particularly the work of Michel Foucault – now played a larger role than 15 years earlier.[6]

Judged by numbers of books and journals published, by the new millennium the discipline had become spectacularly popular, with an ever wider range of historians gravitating towards medical or medically-inflected topics. No unitary style could be identified. But 'eclectic empiricism' gives a flavour of the dominant approach. In the new millennium the histories of learning difficulty and physical disability, child abuse and obesity vie with more traditional topics. In the 1970s and 1980s the nineteenth century and early modern periods attracted more attention than any others. Now increasing numbers of writers engage with twentieth century and near-contemporary topics. However, as we shall see, links between socio-medical and environmental history remain under-developed.[7]

Fifteen years before I began to ponder the histories of environment and disease, there had been a breakthrough in historical epidemiology. Thomas McKeown, a Canadian-born, Irish-educated expert in social medicine, who worked for many years at the University of Birmingham, published a cluster of journals on the nineteenth-century British mortality decline.[8] Sceptical of the achievements of professional medicine – and indifferent throughout his career to criticisms levelled at his own contributions – in 1973 McKeown summarized his findings in *The Modern Rise of Population*. He argued that in late nineteenth century Britain a 'municipal sanitary revolution', a handful of changes in the balance between host and causative microorganisms, and, most important of all, radical improvements in nutrition, had triggered improvements in health.[9] Little wonder that, in his sociological writings, McKeown revealed a career-long obsession with the 'limits of medicine'.[10]

In the 1950s and 1960s there had also been a flurry of activity in what then tended to be called the history of public health. Three books creatively complemented McKeown's research. S.E.Finer, R.A. Lewis and R.S. Lambert published major lives of Edwin Chadwick and Sir John Simon, founding-fathers of Victorian sanitary thinking and the prevention of disease.[11] Finer, Lewis and Lambert identified seminal questions connected with epidemics, conceptions of the transmission of infection and the development of public utilities, notably water supply. Other highly suggestive work around this time derived from economic history, the subject I was studying at the London School of Economics in the early 1970s. E. J. Hobsbawm made a characteristically trenchant contribution to the long-running standard of living debate. He suggested that opposing camps – 'optimists' and 'pessimists' – may have fought themselves to a standstill. Ever larger quantities of quantitative data could be collected, interpreted and haggled over. But to what end? Intriguingly, from my point of view, Hobsbawm believed that greater attention should now be paid to then deeply unfashionable 'qualitative' topics – health and illness and environment.[12]

Differences between quantitative and qualitatively-oriented research in the 1960s and 1970s resonated with much earlier debates between John and Barbara Hammond and the distinguished Cambridge economic historian, Sir John Clapham. The best-selling Hammonds argued that tragically large numbers of working-class inhabitants of new towns had fallen victim to the squalid environments in which they had been forced to live.[13] In the late 1920s they contested Clapham's quantitatively-based assessment of the fortunes of typical members of the working-classes during the first great period of urbanization: these findings, they argued, were too heavily dependent on exclusively statistical data. Clapham acknowledged the force of the point, but doubted whether either optimistic or pessimistic hypotheses could be decisively proven or disproven. The Hammonds accepted that Clapham had clinched the quantitative case but insisted that the social aspect remain open.[14]

What, meanwhile, of the state and status in the early 1970s of what would later come to be known as urban-environmental history? Other things being equal, one would have expected these years to have seen an upsurge in interest in this field. The world oil crisis, pollution, the negative side-effects of rapid economic growth and the unconstrained expansion of world population, generated wide-ranging political debate and an impressive social scientific literature.[15] Contemporary problems invariably shape the questions historians ask about the past. Not in this case. Perhaps the influence of the British arts–science divide, the focus of a heated debate between C.P. Snow and F.R. Leavis in the 1950s, provided a part-explanation.[16] In addition, senior urban and social historians in the 1970s made it clear that environmental and epidemiological research should be left to scientifically-trained specialists.[17] As I would soon discover, things were different in the United States. In the early 1970s a small group of scholars – with Joel Tarr of Carnegie-Mellon University in Pittsburgh in the lead – began to publish on urban-environmental problems in the nineteenth and twentieth century city.[18] The message spread slowly. European and Scandinavian scholars lagged behind. Britain brought up the rear.[19]

Tracing patterns of disease

The first chapter in this book, originally published in 1980, was heavily influenced by McKeown and Hobsbawm. It concentrated on McKeown's hypothesis that a handful of infections – notably scarlet fever and possibly typhus – had entered a late nineteenth century period of decline following a sudden shift in the balance between host and causative microorganism.[20] The chapter also assessed problems associated with annual cause- and age-specific mortality data. McKeown's work had relied on national decennial material and had thrown little light on differentials between town and country, the fortunes of individual urban centres, and different parts of the same locality.[21] I could hardly have guessed that my tentative foray into McKeown territory would generate enough problems to keep me occupied for the next 30 years. Either directly or indirectly, each of the chapters in this book engages with issues first raised in that chapter.

In 1983 I tackled the McKeown typhus hypothesis head-on. (Typhoid provided a kind of control. As McKeown had argued, the decline of the bacterial infection had been closely linked to successive waves of Victorian and Edwardian environmental intervention. Human agency, rather than ecological change, had been decisive.[22])

The existence or otherwise of a change in case-fatality rates proved central to the typhus issue. Cross-cutting between the reports of medical officers of health, the medical press, hospital data, Poor Law records, and the annual cause-specific data provided by the GRO allowed me to construct an index of a wide range of urban disease experiences.[23] The trend seemed to confirm McKeown's theory. However, something different was clearly happening in the urban north-east, where serious outbreaks of the disease continued intermittently to attack poverty-stricken communities. Crucially, in Sunderland and Newcastle in the 1880s as many individuals were failing to survive out of every hundred contracting the infection as in the violently fever-prone aftermath of the Napoleonic Wars, the poverty-plagued 1840s and the final large-scale national epidemic of the 1860s.[24]

Could there be a connection between north-eastern exceptionalism and the natural history of the infection in Ireland? Pools of typhus survived in rural areas in that country and streams of migrants were known to carry the disease into Belfast, Cork and Dublin, before setting sail for England.[25] Another point. In the later nineteenth century the urban north-east received far larger numbers of first-generation Irish than any other part of England. My work on typhus now reminds me of a classic Chinese box puzzle: every problem led on to another of greater evidential complexity. A few years later my conclusions were convincingly challenged by Anne Hardy.[26] However, the exercise deepened my awareness of a cluster of problems first glimpsed in the 1970s – changing nineteenth century conceptions of infectious disease, preventive priorities in the aftermath of the cholera and fever years and subsequent efforts to track and explain cause-specific mortality and morbidity. One other point. The typhus research clarified the depth of pessimism and panic experienced and expressed by earlier nineteenth century social reformers and medical men: at any moment, they feared, the new urban civilization might be decimated by a new outbreak of 'plague-like' infection. As if to fulfil worst expectations, cholera struck in 1831–2, 1848–9, 1854–5 and 1866. Would early and mid-Victorian cities slip back towards the epidemiological misery experienced in the era of the bubonic plague or, at best, the epidemic-ravaged seventeenth and eighteenth centuries?[27]

Even before the shock of the 'final catastrophe' in 1866, described in Chapter 4, attitudes had begun to shift. At meetings of the Epidemiological Society, the Meteorological Society, the Society of Metropolitan Medical Officers and the Sanitary (later Royal Sanitary) Institute, new approaches began to emerge.[28] Progressive health officials in London – and Liverpool – now started to focus on multi-causal explanations of the spread of disease.[29] In the capital reformers emphasized the central importance of effective communication between local medical officers, the General Register Office and the capital-wide Metropolitan Asylums Board (MAB).

This latter organization served as a multi-centre facility for very poor patients – initially paupers – suffering from what were believed to be dangerously infectious conditions.[30] There was a growing consensus that London's preventive system possessed the potential to defeat cholera, typhus and typhoid. Human and animal filth must continue to be regularly removed from ill-ventilated streets and alleys, individuals suffering from dangerous conditions taken to isolation hospitals, and working-class dwellings stricken by infection 'closed down' and declared uninhabitable.[31] (Scandalously little, however, was done to rehouse the exceptionally large numbers thrown out of house and home.[32]) If measures of this kind were carried out in every centre, life in early twentieth century urban Britain might be healthier and happier for every social class. By now, the epidemiological bar was beginning to be raised. Greater attention was paid to conditions which, year in, year out, killed many more people, particularly among the youngest age-groups, than infections like cholera, typhus and typhoid. Morbidity, as well as mortality, were more rigorously monitored. For centuries, working men and women had contracted serious illnesses, recovered and then slowly returned to a kind of health. But physical resilience was invariably compromised. A worker who had recovered from a serious attack of typhoid might never again be able to do a demanding manual job.[33] Knock-on effects could be extreme. Wages declined and lower family take-home pay involved moving further down the housing ladder.[34]

Sub-standard living conditions, and inadequate diet, increased the likelihood of a weakened constitution succumbing to further infection or chronic illness. The only alternatives might be odd-jobbing, street-selling or scavenging. From that narrow ledge, 'dependency' – the workhouse – threatened ominously.[35]

The final third of the nineteenth century also saw increased scrutiny of the spatial incidence of disease. Medical officers charted the ways in which administrative sub-divisions had obscured the precise distribution of poverty, infection and death. The mapping of islands of deprivation in the midst of plenty or relative plenty generated disturbing questions about the maldistribution of wealth – and health – in the greatest and, as many said, the richest city in the world. [36] By the end of the 1870s, we detect the beginnings of an understanding of the processes that might underlie appallingly high levels of mortality from the infections of infancy and childhood: the debate continued into the Edwardian period and the depression-ravaged 1930s.[37] During this period, also, scientists and medical men gradually began to use a wide range of terms – 'poison', 'germ', 'fungus' – to bestow a clearer identity on the minute entities that probably played a central or supportive role in transmitting infection and triggering traumatic outbreaks of disease.[38]

Interrogating this latter theme in the context of the 'final catastrophe' – the cholera epidemic that struck the East End of London in 1866 – Chapter 4 examines the numerous ways in which metropolitan medical officers of health attempted to make conceptual sense of a devastating tragedy. Water lay at the heart of the narrative. Edward Frankland, chemist and unofficial metropolitan water analyst, worked in close collaboration with William Farr, John Simon and John Netten Radcliffe, a pioneering epidemiologist and collaborator of Simon's at the Medical Office of the Privy Council. After numerous investigations, the East London Water Company was condemned 'before the bar of public opinion'. By drawing on sub-standard reserves and pumping cholera into stand-pipes in some of the poorest and most vulnerable parts of the city, it had breached legislation passed a decade and half earlier. The government delivered a muted reprimand and asked the company to behave better in the future. During and after the epidemic, medical officers – and Simon and Farr but not the arch-progressive Radcliffe – hedged their theoretical bets.

A clear majority acknowledged the importance of the 'water factor' but denied that it provided a full explanation. A number of medical officers floated logically irrefutable alternatives. Henry Letheby, Simon's successor as Medical Officer of the City of London, argued that the cholera 'poison' was just as likely to have been spread by the gas supply as by infected water.[39] A clear majority combined a Chadwickian or post-Chadwickian sanitarian stance with selected elements of radical theories first articulated by John Snow and William Budd in the 1850s and early 1860s. Nearly all remained convinced that the ineptitude of local vestries and the sanitary habits of impoverished East End victims themselves played a central role in precipitating the disaster. An anonymous contributor to the *Medical Times and Gazette* asked whether it might not be 'a wise act of humanity ... to say to the local authorities – cleanse your streets and we will relieve [the cholera victims]; but we will send neither money nor wine till the scavenger has gone before us'.[40] And, more ruthlessly, 'pure water, and plenty of it, might save many a gallon of port wine. It would [also] be something to send soap, that the school children of Bethnal-green might get a good wash.'[41]

Modes of epidemiological explanation which directly or indirectly blamed victims of disease for their own misfortunes in the new urban civilization recur in nearly every chapter of this book. Charity came at a price.[42] In 1866 the Queen's Private Secretary announced that the monarch would donate £500 to the Cholera Fund of the Metropolitan Relief and District Visiting Association.[43] Spurred on by Mr and Mrs Gladstone's offer to allow 20 East End orphans to stay on their estate at Hawarden, the Lord Mayor established a Mansion House Cholera Relief Committee.[44] By the end of the first week in August 1866, the charity had spawned 92 local committees helping women and children who had been left without support following the death of an adult bread-winner. When the Mansion House Fund was wound up in mid-November, it was estimated that, together with the London Hospital Cholera Fund, it had raised the enormous sum of £70,000.

But scale of recompense was governed by the stern principles underlying mid-nineteenth charity and moral-sanitarian ideas about the role that the working-classes themselves played in the dissemination of disease. No orphan received funds if his or her parents had earlier been in receipt of parochial relief: claimants of this kind must first seek assistance from the guardians. Nor did boys and girls qualify for charitable help if it could be shown that they were able to live with relatives capable of caring for them.

Children who had lost a mother, but whose father was still 'alive and able to work', were also denied access to relief. Convalescent homes accepting cholera patients were told to demonstrate an identifiable social return in terms of a rapid return to work. 'No greater boon' it was claimed, '[could] be conferred on the poor in sickness than to aid them in the earlier stages of recovery by giving them the means of removal into a purer air'. But they must only be 'maintained' until they were 'strong enough to return to work'.[45] In hard-hit Bethnal Green both the guardians and the vestry stuck rigidly to the rules governing the disbursement of funds as these operated in normal times. Both were put to shame by the spontaneous relief efforts of a minority of socially concerned Anglican clergy, the Sisters of Mercy and *ad hoc* school committees which provided urgently needed food, clothes and hand-outs of cash during a profound epidemic crisis.[46]

Every mid- and later nineteenth century urban centre faced the same problems as the capital. However, as Chapter 5 shows, provincial health bureaucracies prided themselves on the extent to which they had overtaken London in their 'democratic' approach to environmental control and the prevention of disease. Adult and infant death rates, collected on an annual basis by the GRO, provided a broadly accurate picture of improvement, stagnation or deterioration in different parts of the country. Provincial centres prided themselves on the progress they had made and caste the capital in the role of poverty- and illness-ridden laggard. However, to the astonishment of informed observers in Liverpool, Manchester and Glasgow, the facts strongly implied that – despite the existence of vast tracts of poverty and environmental deprivation – London might now be the healthiest city in Britain, or the world.[47] Sometimes, surely, statistics lied?

From the eighteenth century onwards, condescending southern observers had visited Leeds, Sheffield, Birmingham and Manchester and, in the style of colonial explorers or anthropologists, bundled manufacturing centres together into a standardized category labelled the 'new industrial districts'. Following the Municipal Corporations Act every community developed its own sense of constitutional legitimacy and civic pride.[48] New governing bodies had little in common with agencies long concerned with health and environment in the capital. Municipalization spread its wings. Political progressives in later nineteenth century Manchester and Birmingham held to a clear vision of the purpose of urban democracy.[49] Rate-payers must use their vote to confirm possession of a material stake in the city in which they lived and whose services they subsidized. For their part, councils were expected to keep careful watch over sub-committees concerned with public water supply, sewage disposal, housing, health, parks and recreation. London-style 'independency', whereby a group of nominated gentlemen, semi-automatically appointed under ancient charter, went about their business without due scrutiny by an elected city-wide authority, must be eradicated.

This outline simplifies an astonishingly complex picture. For one thing, the capital's own fractious movement for centralizing democratic reform drew partly on metropolitan and partly on provincial traditions and ideologies.[50] The indirectly elected Metropolitan Board of Works (MBW) possessed limited powers, most of them connected with the construction and administration of the main sewage system.[51] When vestries chose to ignore its requests, they found it easy enough to do so. In 1889, to the relief of metropolitan and provincial radicals alike, the endemically corruption-prone MBW was replaced by the London County Council (LCC).[52] However, a list of services and functions excluded from the control of the new body gives an idea of the extent to which 'medieval' traditions survived in the capital into the earlier twentieth century. The LCC had only marginal powers in relation to public water supply, prevention of pollution and what Victorians called the 'purification' of the rivers Thames and Lea, disease control at local level, isolation and hospitalization of infected patients throughout the capital, and reduction of atmospheric pollution.[53]

Pessimistic 'planetary' obsessions

Earlier nineteenth century observers of the urban condition were convinced that overblown new towns and cities would one day sink beneath the weight of their own filth. This catastrophist vision peaked between the early 1830s and the mid-1850s. Sewage poured into inner city wells, streams and rivers: human and animal waste lay as thick as farmyard mud in poverty-stricken alleys. By the 1840s and 1850s Chadwick's plans for the capital, and other urban centres – linking public water supply to sewage disposal – gave birth to the idea of the city as a producing, consuming and waste-intensive organism.[54] This image merged with the notion of flow.[55] Inner city districts would be cleansed and sewage transported to the countryside, where it could be diluted or deodorized and sold to farmers as fertilizer to boost agricultural production. Flow would then be reversed, with cheaper food being transported back to the city. Reduced death rates could generate larger public or private – preferably private – profits.[56]

Blueprints involving two-way flow were only rarely translated into reality. Chapter 6, which marked a change of emphasis in my research interests in the 1990s, with environmental gradually replacing epidemiological concerns, charts the infrastructural history of a range of communities between the early nineteenth and mid-twentieth centuries. It confirms that, between 1850 and 1900, large-scale sewage systems were constructed in every major centre.[57] However, the agricultural dimension of the waste-transporting and disposing process failed to yield the benefits that had been over-optimistically attributed to it. How, at the level of everyday economics, could a farmer in the hinterland of mid-nineteenth century Leeds use – or pay for? – the vast volumes of waste daily offered to him under a sewage disposal scheme?

This topic has received less attention in Britain than the United States, where, from the early 1970s onwards, urban-environmental

historians undertook pioneering research into the scale and typology
– and attempts to minimize the impact – of city-based pollution, the
politics of waste disposal, the strengths and weaknesses of proposed
infrastructural solutions and the strains placed on town–country
relations by a failure to neutralize ever larger volumes of noxious by-
products. The search for an 'ultimate sink' – Joel Tarr's term –
gained wide currency.[58] The phrase referred to a place in nature – did
it, could it ever exist? – where waste would be rendered harmless
and, if civil and sanitary engineers found viable solutions,
transformed into fertilizer. The quest for an 'ultimate sink' was
closely linked to the idea of the transposition of pollution problems.
Inter-communal conflict, triggered by the alleviation of one centre's
difficulties at the expense of another's, indicated the ways in which
large-scale urbanization generated effects that lacked a clear spatial
identity – or, in terms of the creation of an alleged nuisance – legal
culpability.[59] Transposition problems also highlighted the inter-
relatedness of every process in nature and 'second nature', generating
and slowly shaping linked bodies of post-sanitarian, environmental
and ecological thought.[60]

A river polluted by the waste of a town upstream endangered the
water supply and welfare of communities lower down: smoky factory
chimneys and domestic hearths undermined health – particularly
among the very young and the elderly – for miles around.[61]
Landowners, tenant farmers and millers dependent on an
unhampered and relatively clean flow of water joined battle with
large towns. So did smaller localities. Pigmies confronted giants.
Appealing to the powerful doctrine of local self-government,
expanding municipalities and smaller locations demanded freedom
both to run their own affairs without interference from central state
bureaucracies and without being subjected to bullying tactics by
over-bearing towns.[62] For their part, powerful big-city councillors
claimed that the burden of responsibility for the health of large
populations must override 'privileged' demands for amenity on the
part of villages, market towns and landowners.

A combination of the failure to find an 'ultimate sink' and the
problem of transposition changed the manner in which medical

officers and growing numbers of scientists with a specialized interest in reducing pollution conceptualized the ways in which infections spread from one community to another and relationships between town and country in an ever more heavily urbanized society. During the final 20 years of the nineteenth century, the influence of long imbedded miasmatic orthodoxy and its derivatives entered a period of terminal decline. A cluster of complementary disciplines came to the fore and merged with selected elements of sanitarian orthodoxy to generate new approaches to the prevention of disease.[63] This period, between the 1870s and the outbreak of World War I, saw a raising of both the environmental and the epidemiological bars: the two processes went hand-in-hand.

As Chapter 6 shows, water, both for drinking, industrial and commercial uses and transporting waste away from town centres, had been central to reformist thinking between the 1830s and the 1870s. From the 1870s onwards, however, research into the impact of contaminated air on human health produced a new form of anxiety and gave rise to numerous unsuccessful attempts to introduce preventive legislation.[64] My interest in this topic was originally triggered in the early 1970s following a chance reading of half a paragraph in a textbook by the distinguished economic historian Sidney Checkland. Checkland described the impact of highly noxious white dust produced by mid-nineteenth alkali works in St Helens – the town where these words are being written. Tenant farmers stumbled through withered crops. Cattle gasped for breath and woodland was reduced to dismal clumps of gnarled branches and roots.[65] These sombre images stayed with me and, much later, drew me towards a related and at that time under-explored topic – the nature, impact and cultural ramifications of atmospheric pollution, produced by thousands on thousands of domestic hearths. Without realizing it, I had stumbled into the heart of a late nineteenth century London fog.[66]

Choking smoke had been an unnerving seasonal presence in towns since mid-century. Twenty years on, the position had become critical. Meteorologists and 'fog specialists' now realized that hundreds of thousands of hearths, particularly in ever-expanding suburbia, might pose a more serious threat to health and amenity than uncontrolled factory stacks. Not only, as Chapters 7 and 8 show, did the smoke problem encourage epidemiologists to reassess the impact of atmospheric pollution on human health, and conclude that, at its worst, a 'yellow' or 'gritty' London fog might account for as many deaths as the cholera epidemic of 1854–5. It also brought environmentalists and meteorologists into closer proximity with the everyday life-and-death problems encountered by the poor and desperately poor. A five-day fog-induced commercial and industrial near-close-down in a large city involved significant loss of income, particularly among the casually employed. Adverse atmospheric conditions were invariably accompanied by icy anti-cyclonic weather. Desperate economic conditions, associated with loss of work attributable to the fog-generated freezing of everyday commercial life, led to a reduction in expenditure on fuel: intense cold increased the incidence of life-threatening bronchial and general respiratory disease.[67] Direct and indirect side-effects were listed – and shakily quantified – by atmospheric observers, notably the influential late nineteenth century 'fog expert', the aristocratic Francis (Rollo) Russell.[68]

The discovery of the perils of unregulated atmospheric pollution coincided with the development of environmentally-rooted styles of analysis directed at a reconceptualization of relationships between human health and the side-effects of mass urbanization. These were attributed to greatly increased production and consumption and what were now more widely deemed 'backward' and 'dirty' factory and workshop methods. At the same time – the final 30 years of the nineteenth century – styles of anti-urban thinking which had been present in the earlier nineteenth century, and which shaped the world-view of historians like John and Barbara Hammond, gained increased momentum.

There might be evidence to the contrary – declining death-rates, slowly improving housing conditions and cleaner streets. But this did little to reduce the intensity of *fin de siecle* pessimism. At an extreme, a spectrum of related and intertwined discourses, heavily influenced by and interacting with social Darwinism, fear of national race degeneration, and an often mistaken belief in the inevitability of absolute, rather than relative and-or regional-cum-sectoral economic decline, drew on the ills of the city as a scapegoat for a range of woes that were often only distantly related to what was actually happening in real urban milieux.[69] The dark and depressing metropolitan fog epidemic between the 1870s and the Edwardian era reinforced these fears and gave rise to the belief that towns, industries and households had been irresponsibly profligate in their use of finite energy resources.

W.S. Jevons's *The Coal Question*, published in 1866, the same year as the final major British cholera epidemic, became a seminal text.[70] Intense debate continued for more than 30 years, complemented and reinforced by a more extreme form of anti-urbanism than had first come to the fore in the early and mid-nineteenth century. By the 1880s there was a widespread belief that only some kind of ill-defined mass 'return to the country' might save Britain from an 'arctic' future. Unless a solution were to be rapidly found, a greatly diminished population would be forced to endure a primitive existence amid the ruins of what had once been the most advanced urban-industrial civilization the world had ever seen. Entropic images proved irresistible to social and cultural pessimists: urban society – perhaps, even, the planet – might be prematurely 'running down'.[71]

Specialist knowledge concerned with the pollution of air and water now finally and decisively defined itself over and against post-Chadwickian sanitarianism. As panicked comment in Chapter 7 reveals, increasing numbers of cultural critics and social reformers became obsessed by the problem of the city, but now as a metaphor for global crisis as well as cultural and race decline. At the same time, leading scientists – those working on the pollution of rivers and water supplies, with Edward Frankland in the lead and Angus Smith pre-eminent in the struggle against smoke – hoped against hope that specialist knowledge might one day feed into tougher legislative action.[72] Nevertheless, as the overview in Chapter 6 shows, the translation of new knowledge into effective panaceas was long resisted by powerful manufacturing and municipal interest-groups. The half century between 1900 and the terrifying London smog of

1952 witnessed repeated parliamentary failure, or disinclination, effectively to engage with pollution problems first identified between 1870 and 1914.[73] After the passing of the Clean Air Act in 1956, it was nearly a decade before British urban-industrial skies became consistently clearer. Cleaning up rivers advanced in an even more leisurely manner. As late as 1945 legislative and administrative control remained rudimentary: the introduction of effective and coordinated action against pollution attributable to sewage and industrial effluent required many more years of public, parliamentary and ministerial action.[74] During each sub-period enforcement criteria lagged behind progressive scientific consensus.

Decoding environmental discourses

The final two chapters trace recurring theoretical and conceptual themes that have been explicitly or implicitly present in every chapter of the book and follows them into the near-present. As every historian knows, this can be dangerous. Over-linear narratives exaggerate continuities at the expense of disjunctions in ideological, scientific and discursive representation and change. Nevertheless, Chapter 9 identifies the survival of passionate pro-rural – and potently anti-urban – tendencies in later twentieth century Britain, similar to but less rhetorically strident than the ideas and attitudes that accompanied and intensified generalized late nineteenth century pessimism and despair. Like their predecessors, near-contemporary and early twenty first century champions of the virtues of the countryside have rarely engaged with specific conditions in specific towns, or with the *places* that make up urban localities that in turn generate their own distinctive traditions, cultures, and solutions to urban-based or regional problems.[75] The marginalization of suburbia continues to ensure over-reliance on an over-simplified and outmoded dichotomy between town and country. A British – more accurately, Anglocentric – yearning for a rural alternative to city life endures.

Finally, there is the issue of environmental justice, a theme subtextually present in every chapter in this book but rarely, I hope, in what is here called the 'wide spectrum' form that has become increasingly popular among American scholars.[76] This latter approach draws on and uses the past to validate and strengthen contemporary political activism. Chapter 9 juxtaposes Dolores Greenberg's undoubtedly persuasive 'wide spectrum' article on historical aspects of environmental justice and protest in New York City against Harold Platt's account of Jane Addams's reformist activities in early twentieth century Chicago. I argue that Platt's approach makes adjustments and qualifications central to meaningful interpretation of ideologies and aims strikingly similar to but at the same time radically different from early twenty first century experience.[77] This is less a plea to go back to writing about the past in the language of actors with whom the historian has become intimately involved: that way lies descriptivism, antiquarianism – and irrelevance. But when nineteenth century discourses give too much ground to ideas and values that rose to prominence in the later twentieth century, something – perhaps a great deal – is lost.

The reasons are clear. The emergence and trajectory of the idea of pollution in the nineteenth and earlier twentieth centuries – and the cognitive and scientific networks of which it became a part – is now much more thoroughly understood than was the case two or three decades ago.[78] But not so 'environment' or environmentalism.[79] In the United States, continental Europe and Britain the years between the 1870s and the outbreak of World War I witnessed the emergence of concepts and theories that would in the near future become central to new ways of conceptualizing relationships between *homo sapiens*, nature and 'second nature'.[80] However, as nearly every chapter in this book suggests, in that same period this still novel bundle of ideas and hypotheses remained partially and confusingly obscured beneath an overlay of seemingly indefinitely flexible post-sanitarian doctrine and discourse. Any number of later nineteenth and early twentieth century epidemiologists, medical men and public health reformers continued to communicate their ideas in ways that had less to do with the centrality of a deep interaction and interpenetration between humans and their environments than repeatedly modified ways of reconstructing and moralizing *place* – street, court, alley, house, room, stairwell.

James Winter has expressed the same idea in the following, illuminating, terms. 'In the nineteenth century, connotations would have been closer to the etymological roots of *environment:* the country around, the neighbourhood, the environs, the stretch of topography that gave definition to a place, one's own surroundings.'[81] These deeply imbedded perceptions and categorizations and the health-oriented panaceas with which they were associated, continued to be shaped by a largely taken-for-granted world-view shaped by fixed ideas of class and caste, religion, deference and charity. The words that reformers used still seem alien to us and require close reading and decoding on their own terms rather than within the context of the countless environmental and epidemiological concerns of the early twenty first century.

In this kind of work, there is no option but to use our own linguistic resources. How else to interpret and communicate the character and uniqueness of the periods and topics which we have long pondered and now seek to explain? The chapters in this book try to make sense of the still often puzzling words and discourses used by public health reformers when they described and – the progressives among them – sought to reduce the scale and persistence of death, debilitated survival and environmental threat and deprivation in the nineteenth and twentieth century city.

CHAPTER 2

DEATH AND SURVIVAL IN THE CITY: APPROACHES TO THE HISTORY OF DISEASE

Disciplinary dilemmas and possibilities

Now that the debate about the standard of living during the first half of the nineteenth century appears to have entered a relatively quiescent phase, historians have begun to turn their attention towards the more elusive concept of the quality of life.[1] The incidence of fatal and non-fatal disease is clearly central to research of this type and so, too, is a delineation of the physical context in which infections have flourished and in which those who have been afflicted by them have lived. Although there has been a tendency to underestimate the ferocity of epidemics in rural areas in the period after about 1750, historians working on disease in the modern period are inevitably most usually concerned with processes which are specifically urban in character. And urban historians, especially those interested in such topics as the development of utilities, the growth of administrative bureaucracies or the spatial segregation and different life experiences of the classes, can undoubtedly benefit from a knowledge of patterns of infection in the past.

There are, in fact, a number of wholly unforced and fruitful connections to be made between urban history and the history of disease. It would also seem reasonable to assume that the historian of disease and the urban historian who makes use of selected epidemiological material would gain from a close acquaintanceship with the venerable discipline of the history of medicine. But, paradoxical though it may seem, historians of medicine have in fact written remarkably little about the actual incidence and mass experience of disease in history. Why this should be so (why, that is, the history of medicine should have remained largely indifferent to what would seem to be a crucial field of inquiry) is an intriguing and complicated question: and an explanation of this historiographical peculiarity, even the abbreviated account offered in the introduction to this chapter, should reveal something of the intellectual pedigree and current state of the history of disease.

The failure to confront the 'hard facts' of disease in the past is partly explicable in terms of the history of medicine itself – a discipline which has traditionally been the province of those whose main interests have been in the evolution of medical theories and practice rather than in relationships between medicine, disease and society at large. It is a style of history which has been more concerned with the development of diagnosis and therapy, of sub-disciplines and specialisms – anatomy, physiology, surgery, anaesthesia, paediatrics, psychiatry and so on – than with the great mass of people in whom ill-health has, as it were, been physically and psychically located. Medical history, like all history, has also been strongly influenced by current preoccupations. Therapies which cannot be shown to have contributed to an ever more effective body of medical expertise have been largely ignored. And with a few exceptions – the very different work, for example, of Michel Foucault and Brian Abel-Smith[2] – the institutional history of hospitals and of hospitalization has been dominated by assumptions that are rooted in the here-and-now. Improvements in medical practice and education have, according to this view, been made to flow in a linear and predetermined manner from what has gone before, and to lead on to what is known to have followed.

It is not simply that discontinuities have remained unclear as a result of this approach: but, more seriously, that the most fundamental of all historical processes, that of change, has been tacitly excluded. Nevertheless, a small number of scholars have over the years fashioned a rather different type of medical history. Erwin Ackerknecht has propounded challenging hypotheses about connections between a prevailing political climate and dominant theories as to the transmission of disease:[3] the late George Rosen has charted the long-term behaviour of the major European infections and the ways in which medical and political bureaucracies have reacted to the threat of epidemics:[4] and Joseph Needham, in his magisterial researches into the history of East Asian science and medicine, has challenged numerous Whiggish and Eurocentric orthodoxies.[5]

More recently, a growing though still small number of social, political and urban historians have been engaged upon work on the historical incidence of disease and the ways in which it has been perceived and treated. In his studies of the plague in the city states of Italy, Carlo Ciplolla has indicated how individual communities organized themselves against epidemics and the extent to which economic self-interest determined which from among a range of competing theories of disease was the most likely to be adopted by particular social groups.[6] In *Religion and the Decline of Magic* Keith Thomas has demonstrated how historians may make use of anthropological concepts to shed light on differences between specialist and popular images of therapy and disease.[7]

In a number of provocative journals, in which he has applied contemporary findings in epidemiology and the food sciences to reconstituted demographic data of the type assembled by the Cambridge Group for the History of Population and Social Structure, Andrew Appleby has sought to disentangle the relative contributions of malnutrition and infection to high levels of mortality in preindustrial society.[8] Phillipe Ariés and Ivan Illich, the latter in his polemical *Medical Nemesis* which sparked off a small-scale debate within the medical profession, have traced changing attitudes towards suffering and death.[9] In the field of nineteenth-century studies, with which this chapter is primarily concerned, three pioneering historians, Sidney Finer and R. A. Lewis in their complementary studies of Edwin Chadwick, and R. S. Lambert in his seminal work on John Simon, have described the political and environmental assumptions of the vanguard of the first national campaign for the improvement of public health in an industrial society.[10]

There has as yet, however, been little detailed research into the explicitly quantitative incidence of disease, or of specific infections, in the late eighteenth and nineteenth centuries.[11] It may be the case, of course, that social and economic historians have tended to be intimidated by the technical demands posed by medical history and, in this respect, it can hardly be a matter of chance that the standard journals by Thomas McKeown and his colleagues at the University of Birmingham on changes in aggregate mortality between the later eighteenth and mid-twentieth centuries should have been written by specialists in social medicine.[12] But this is an argument which cuts both ways. It is hardly surprising that social and urban historians venturing into medical territory should feel that their hypotheses are likely to be demolished by the medical expert. But it may also be the case that researchers whose primary training has been medical will over-simplify findings in social and economic history.

The remainder of this chapter will examine ways in which urban and social historians may set about tackling topics which were, until quite recently, assumed to lie exclusively within the domain of the research worker blessed with a specialist medical background. A brief comment on the quality of the statistical data relating to infectious disease in the nineteenth century is followed by an account of how such evidence may be made to throw light on otherwise elusive aspects of environmental change. The ensuing discussion of the variables which must enter into any attempt to clarify the changing behaviour of infections with the passage of time leads into a critique of what is here loosely defined as 'microorganic determinism' – the hypothesis that shifts in mortality due to a number of demographically important diseases have been less powerfully influenced by medical intervention or by programmes of urban reform than by purportedly 'random' biological and-or ecological modifications. The chapter concludes with some remarks on recent work in the social and political interpretation of epidemics during the nineteenth century.

Decoding deceptive sources

The fundamental source material for the historian of disease in the nineteenth century, the annual and decennial *Reports* of the Registrar-General, must be approached with a high degree of caution and scepticism. The ever-changing categorization of disease during the first 20 years or so of registration, and the failure to achieve a convincing differentiation between several of the most important infections until after mid-century, involves the research worker in a constant battle to ensure that like is being compared with like. To take a single and representative example: the symptomologically similar but etiologically quite distinct infections of typhus and typhoid only came to be reliably differentiated from one another in the Registrar's *Reports* in the late 1860s. In this, as in several comparable instances, the historian is forced to seek out other categories of evidence which may clarify the epidemiological nuances obscured by the medically misleading aggregates contained in the official returns. Thus in London in the mid-nineteenth century, and many of the examples in this chapter will be based on the epidemiological experience of the capital, progressive medical men at the Fever Hospital in Islington as well as a number of well-informed medical officers of health made calculations of what they believed to have been the approximate incidence of the two diseases from the late 1840s onwards.[13]

Another weakness of the registration material is that it fails throughout the nineteenth century to make allowance for patients whose 'normal place of residence' was deemed to be in district A but who actually died in a hospital or public institution in district B. It is extremely difficult to make adjustments for distortions of this type in the early post-registration period. But from about 1870 onwards it becomes increasingly feasible to cross-check the Registrar's *Reports* against the admissions registers of those public hospitals which were beginning to accept larger numbers of working-class patients, and thus to 'redistribute' deaths from one district to another.[14]

It should be noted, however, that this juggling with data at district level – and most urban historians will inevitably be more

interested in differentials within large urban areas than in crude
aggregates for the community as a whole – can be exceptionally
time-consuming. The results, that is, do not always seem to justify
the very large numbers of calculations which have to be undertaken
to construct a corrected, cause-specific district mortality schedule.
Yet probably the most debilitating shortcoming of all is that the
registration material fails to provide an indication of the incidence of
non-fatal illness. It hardly needs emphasizing that, in the almost
total absence of unemployment benefit and minimal health care, a
serious bout of illness affected wage-earners and their dependants in a
number of debilitating ways. Lengthy periods of unemployment led
to a reduction of income available for rent and food, with the result
that families were forced to move to cheaper and less healthy
accommodation and to purchase smaller quantities of less nutritious
food.[15] Lower intakes of food weakened both the sufferer's resistance
to secondary infection and the general level of health of the family as a
whole. Illness bred poverty: increased poverty yet further eroded
resistance to fatal infection.

It is considerably easier to outline the impact of morbidity than to
give it an accurate quantitative expression. In the period before about
1870 case fatality rates derived from the records of the small number
of hospitals which accepted substantial numbers of working-class
patients may be applied to data in the Registrar's *Reports*, but care
must, of course, be taken to assess both the typicality of the hospital
catchment area and the size of the intake in relation to the non-
hospitalized population. For the period after 1870, case fatality rates
for specific infections in large towns are more fully documented in the
reports of medical officers of health and an increasingly authoritative
epidemiological literature. Providing, then, that sufficient attention
is given to the weaknesses and ambiguities of the official registration
material, and especially to the vagaries of cause-specific mortality at
district level, it should be possible to arrive at moderately reliable
estimates of mortality and morbidity for individual infections from
about mid-century onwards. In addition to revealing the
epidemiological profile of a given urban community, and of its
component sub-communities, mortality and morbidity figures may

also be used to assess the scale of pollution in the period before environmental deterioration came to be monitored through independent indicators.

The value of retrospective environmental assessment of this type may be more fully appreciated in the context of the impressive range of qualitative evidence, dating from the 1820s onwards, which shows that town-dwellers from very nearly every social class were fully alive to the newly emergent dangers of pollution. Dominant medical orthodoxies did not, of course, acknowledge that disease such as cholera and typhoid were principally spread via the mass distribution of unsafe water, but this did not inhibit contemporaries from being aware of and protesting against the widespread despoliation of the natural world, and it is, in fact, during the period between about 1820 and 1840 that the word 'environment' first takes on its distinctively modern meaning. It was during this period, also, that public controversy about what are now known as 'environmental problems' – the impact, for example of river pollution on income derived from fishing in the Thames in the late 1820s, or of massive chemical fall-out over the residential districts of St Helens in the 1850s – became unprecedentedly intense.[16]

This awareness of the undesirable side-effects of industrialization and urbanization spread rapidly, yet the effectiveness of the protests of those who condemned the baleful effects of uncontrolled pollution on drinking water or on the saleability of vegetables grown on allotments backing on to factories was necessarily dependent upon impressions which were highly subjective. Industrialists, local authorities and the owners of urban utilities were therefore well placed to argue that a particular instance of pollution had not in fact taken place: to admit that it had taken place but to disclaim responsibility for it: or to accept responsibility but deny that there was a proven medical connection between an alleged incident and increased mortality from a specific cause. Individual crusaders might declaim against the dangers of pollution but the miasmatic theory of disease dictated that those who contended that there was a link between, for example, a polluted river and a wider-ranging outbreak of typhoid or cholera, were usually outgunned.

In our own time, of course, scientists and administrative bureaucracies have access to indicators which enable them to monitor levels of pollution and of diseases which are known to be heavily influenced by particular types of environmental change. The historian of disease, though, is in a less fortunate position and is seriously restricted by the weaknesses of the available evidence – especially the absence, until about the final quarter of the nineteenth century, of any kind of reliable and meaningful environmental series.[17] Since, however, it is now indisputably established that particular infections are invariably associated with particular types of pollution, cause-specific mortality data may be used to yield information about the gravity of such pollution during the nineteenth century. In this sense, rising mortality from cholera, dysentery, diarrhoea and typhoid from the 1840s onwards confirms the validity of the claims of those who campaigned against the unconstrained pollution of the water environment at that time. An analogous but, because of the continuing haziness of Victorian medical categorization, probably a less decisive association may also be posited between what contemporary medical men termed 'diseases of the lungs and chest' and rising levels of atmospheric pollution.

Exploring complex causalities

An explanation of the changing behaviour of a given infection over time involves consideration of a number of social, economic and environmental factors. The availability and reliability of evidence on the most important of these variables for the historian of the nineteenth-century city – population densities, rates of migration, changing levels of *per capita* income and associated levels of nutrition – will now be briefly examined. Since the mode of transmission of the (in quantitative terms) most important diseases in the period under review was predominantly air-borne, mortality and morbidity were decisively influenced by levels of over-crowding. There is now a growing body of literature on this topic as well as on the strengths and weaknesses of the various indices, whether of persons per acre, per house or per room, by which contemporaries attempted to measure population densities.[18] As for migration, the reactivation of epidemic diseases which were transmitted through person-to-person contact or via an insect vector, rather than through an intermediate environment, were frequently sparked off by the arrival of infected individuals into a susceptible population. The precise dynamics of epidemics of this type are more likely to be elucidated by charting sudden and relatively small-scale inter-urban movements, especially those undertaken by the very poor during periods of acute economic distress, than by computing the more conventional net inter-county rates from the *Census* material. The scale and impact of these often socially disruptive migrations may sometimes be partially recovered by exploiting the archives of those large urban hospitals which accepted the poorest of the poor and recorded either their place of birth or their 'normal place of residence'.[19]

The actual death-toll exacted by the individual epidemic was in many instances affected by standards of living and levels of nutrition. Changing *per capita* income, the proportion of income spent on food, its quantity and quality, and when such information finally becomes available, probable *per capita* intakes of calories – all these are essential, though all too often elusive, determinants of nutritional change.[20] Once assembled, material of this type must be interpreted in the light of what is definitively established as to the impact of nutrition on the individual infection – and this is a complex and highly contentious field. (There is, for example, still no absolute agreement as to the precise effect of marginally improved diet on the incidence of typhus in the nineteenth and the twentieth centuries.[21]) A further determinant of the incidence of infectious disease is how people live, their customs and their patterns of behaviour. From this perspective, a crucial question currently facing historians of disease is whether, beginning in the late eighteenth century, it is possible to identify a slow but irreversible sea-change in attitudes towards personal cleanliness: and, a related issue, how much this as yet underdocumented transformation may have contributed to the long-term decline of such infections as cholera, typhus, typhoid and infant diarrhoea.

Statistics relating to the consumption of water for domestic purposes, vital to any systematic examination of changing patterns of communal hygiene, were studiously collected throughout the nineteenth century. But material on regional increases in the consumption of soap, which may have hastened the eradication of the 'dirt diseases', is sparse. So, too, is quantitative and qualitative evidence which might confirm the hypothesis that the mass introduction of cotton clothing was inimical to the louse population which had for so long sustained the ferocity of epidemic typhus. Nor, to complete this catalogue of material for a rigorous account of hygiene in history, is much yet known about the numbers, and the spatial and social distribution of baths, washbasins and water-closets in the new urban areas.[22]

Economic, social and behavioural variables should not, of course, be artificially abstracted from their larger environmental context. There are, broadly speaking, two aspects of the environment which have an important bearing upon infectious disease among humans: the external environment, comprising the natural world, man-made artefacts and the technologies, for the supply of water and the disposal of sewage and waste, with which urban man has sought to minimize filth and infection: and the internal or domestic 'micro-environment', comprising the contents and arrangement of the individual dwelling, the method of conserving food and drink, and the distance between areas used, on the one hand for living and eating and, on the other, for the short-term storage of waste. Although it has not yet been fully tested against the experience of any single nineteenth century urban community, the hypothesis that it was primarily the modification of the external environment between about the mid-1840s and 1870 which precipitated the decline in diseases of the faecal-oral route, notably typhoid and cholera, will probably be found to be substantially correct.[23]

The improvement of the domestic 'micro-environment', on the other hand, only got under way during the first decade of the twentieth century when infant mortality, which the late George Rosen has called 'one of the most sensitive indicators' of the quality of community health, finally began to decline to levels which may be meaningfully compared with those in the developed world today.[24] This amelioration, which made an important impact on the infections of

infancy and childhood (and particularly on infant diarrhoea) has not yet
been at all adequately explained, although it is reasonable to suggest
that it could not have occurred without continuing increases in *per
capita* income, a slowly improving supply of public housing and
greater public awareness of the germ theory of disease.

'Random' ecological change?

And yet the behaviour of a number of infections remains elusive and
apparently unrelated to socio-economic or environmental change.
There has therefore been a growing tendency in recent years,
supported by such historians as Braudel, Henry and Chambers, to
explain epidemiological history – and by extension, the history of
population – in terms of 'random' biological and ecological
transformations.[25] This emergent 'microorganic determinism', a
complement to the geographical and climatic determinism which
have proven so attractive to French historians, and particularly to the
Annales school, presents man as merely one among a multitude of
different types of life on this planet, potentially at the mercy of
autonomous change in the ecologies of the bacteria, viruses and
insect vectors which cause disease among humans. Insofar as it
implies the termination of the absolute supremacy of *homo sapiens*
both in nature and in history, and thus devotes more attention, in the
style of the pioneering virologist MacFarlane Burnet, to the natural
history of microorganic life *per se*, this is a potentially exciting
enterprise.[26] But, in its currently over-generalized form it may, as
Paul Slack has noted, merely serve as a convenient though
unilluminating escape-route for historians whose other explanatory
schema have proven inadequate.[27]

The conception of an 'autonomous' change in the nature of a
disease is itself exceedingly complex for, depending upon the
characteristics of the infection, a very large number of factors and-or
interactions between factors may be involved. These may include a
shift in the toxicity or invasiveness of the microorganism, a sudden
environmental or climatic modification exerting a dramatic effect on
the bioecology of bacteria outside the human body, or a disturbance

in the insect populations which transmit infections to humans. One technique of deciding whether the virulence of an infective micro-organism may have changed – in the manner in which, according to McKeown and Record, the haemolytic streptococcus responsible for scarlet fever changed during the nineteenth century[28] – is to compare case fatality rates when mortality from the disease is high with comparable rates when mortality has undergone a large and rapid reduction. If such comparisons reveal substantial differentials there will be good grounds for exploring the possibility that biological and ecological factors may have played a dominant role. But, if the difference between the two rates is either small or non-existent, behavioural change is likely to be more satisfactorily explained in environmental or socio-economic terms.

Certainly, as ecologically complex a disease as typhus which several writers, over a long period of time, have believed to have been at least partly affected by sudden 'autonomous' changes in virulence, does not in fact display significant intertemporal differentials in case fatality when the large-scale British epidemics of the 1830s and 1860s are compared with small-scale outbreaks during the later nineteenth century.[29] In this case, it is the highly unpredictable long-term periodicity of the disease, its 'long swings', and the nature of the inter-epidemic reservoirs of infections – how the disease manages to preserve itself, as it were, between its recrudescences among human populations – which will probably eventually provide a degree of insight into short-term behavioural change. These comments should not be interpreted as a dismissal of what has here been described as 'microorganic determinism' but rather as an indication that the 'natural history' of a disease is invariably highly complex, and that the major infections which have afflicted European society in modern times will only be fully understood through the application of models which accommodate specific biological and ecological variables. These models will not be easy to construct since they will demand that the historian be acquainted not only with the fundamentals of medicine and bacteriology, but also with aspects of bioecology, parasitology, immunology and the food sciences.

There is, however, no reason why work of this type should precede research into the political and social implications of epidemics during the nineteenth century. Indeed, the two enterprises – the epidemiological and the socio-political – can, and in my view should, be carried on together. Following Asa Briggs' seminal contribution, there has been a steady growth in the number of books, articles and theses devoted to the interpretation of disease and, more particularly, of cholera in the nineteenth century.[30] This body of work has, *inter alia*, documented contradictions between medical and lay ideas on the nature of infection and has shown that sections of the working class believed that cholera epidemics were deliberately spread by Malthusians, seeking to thin out the ranks of the poor, and by medical men eager to obtain supplies of bodies for *post-mortem* dissection.[31] In Britain, in contrast to several European countries, rioting associated with cholera seems only rarely to have interacted and fused with deeper political discontent. Indeed, despite the futility and counter-productiveness of the preventive and therapeutic measures to which they lent their support, both central government and the ruling elites in the hardest hit of the localities appear to have weathered successive visitations with remarkable resilience. We now have monographs on aspects of the epidemiological and social history of cholera in nineteenth century Britain, Russia, France and the United States.[32] The next priority is a genuinely comparative study which would attempt to explain differential reactions to the pandemic in terms of diverse political, institutional and religious structures.

Yet it would be disappointing if future work were to be concentrated on cholera to the exclusion of other, less dramatic, but, in terms of their contribution to aggregate mortality, more important diseases such as tuberculosis, smallpox and the infections of childhood. A distinction may perhaps be drawn between diseases such as cholera, typhus and smallpox, which were traumatic in terms of their observable symptoms and therefore highly visible to large sections of the population, and others, such as tuberculosis and typhoid, the symptoms of which were considerably less conspicuous. The range of provocative questions which might be asked of a highly visible disease such as typhus is very wide – to take just one example, it would be intriguing to know whether and to what extent the large-scale epidemics of the later 1830s and the later 1840s reinforced existing prejudice against newly arrived Irish immigrants in the larger urban areas.

The less sensational diseases will probably generate a different set of questions – whether, for example, it is possible to make a hard-and-fast distinction between the social impact of epidemic and endemic infections in history, how and approximately when endemic diseases ceased to be accepted and suffered as part of the natural order of things, the range of treatments (or pseudo-treatments), 'folk' as well as medical, which were available to different social classes, and how non-fatal illness among infants and children was nursed in the individual home. The theoretical and empirical implications of some of these questions are beginning to be confronted by social historians of medicine.[33] The aim of the present chapter has been to argue that the enduring themes of disease, survival and death should now also be taken up and creatively investigated by urban historians.

CHAPTER 3

EVALUATING THE SANITARY REVOLUTION: TYPHUS AND TYPHOID IN LONDON, 1851–1900

Historical paths of infection

From the sixteenth century typhus and typhoid caused calamitous suffering among European communities.[1] Epidemic typhus swept through towns and villages during periods of warfare and famine: typhoid struck more insidiously whenever and wherever infected water or rotten food were consumed. The two diseases, invariably and erroneously conflated by medical men, were, together with smallpox and the infections of childhood, pre-eminent among those post-plague causes of death which kept mortality at such continuingly high levels between the later seventeenth and the early nineteenth centuries.[2]

Very little is known in precise terms about aggregate mortality from the two diseases in eighteenth-century England but, in the case of typhus, it seems likely that the benefits gained from the alleviation of famine conditions were counterbalanced by the onset of urbanization and by the concentration of unprecedentedly large numbers of the very poor into overcrowded homes and public institutions. Popular terminology – 'jail fever', for example – indicates a correspondence between the emergence of the disease as a 'social problem' and the growth, from the mid-eighteenth century onwards, of agencies – hospitals, workhouses, houses of correction, prisons, asylums – committed, as recent scholarship has begun to demonstrate, to the management and 'treatment' not only of the sick but also of the deviant and the straightforwardly poverty-stricken.[3]

The history of typhoid during the eighteenth century is even more obscure than that of typhus, but it is probable that the growth of population in towns and the increased scale of facilities for the supply of water and food led to high levels of mortality from the disease. The village, or closed community, which drew its water from the same polluted stream or well year after year could expect to lose a fixed proportion of its population every summer and autumn; and, in towns, where techniques of water purification were either unknown or only crudely applied, epidemics were likely to be more widely disseminated.[4] Both diseases continued to thrive in the nineteenth century. Country and capital were severely afflicted by typhus in 1801, 1816–19, 1837–8 and 1846–7, when the pressure of war and demobilization, extreme poverty and uncontrolled Irish immigration provided an ideal environment for the spread of the infection.[5] Death from typhoid at this time was more likely to occur as a result of a regular annual endemic cycle than during an epidemic onslaught, but mortality in urban regions, like that from other water-associated infections such as dysentery, diarrhoea and cholera, nevertheless reached very high levels.

After mid-century, however, mortality from typhus and typhoid began its final decline, leading to a very great alleviation in human suffering – mainly though not exclusively concentrated among the poor – and also contributing to continued demographic growth.[6] Although it is unwise to isolate the quantitative from the experiential in the social history of disease, this chapter will address itself primarily to the question of why it was that typhus and typhoid, which destroyed so many lives between the sixteenth and the mid-nineteenth centuries in England, should, by the early twentieth, have been claiming so few. If demographic questions of this kind are to be satisfactorily settled, it might be argued that the historian should examine a disease, and particularly as ecologically complex an infection as typhus, for a period of a century or more, in order to reveal the changing relationship between vector, host and environment, and also to chart the complex rhythms of dormancy and recrudescence.

However, there is also a strong case for tracing the natural history of an infection over a much shorter period, and in a deliberately delimited geographical area. This latter approach makes it possible to juxtapose the regional against the national pattern; to undertake a detailed analysis of the final phase of an epidemiological downswing; and to analyse concepts which have traditionally dominated discussion of 'fever' and its demographic significance. Each of these aspects is explored in this chapter, beginning with a brief account of the principal characteristics of typhus and typhoid, and an explanation of the inability of so many medical practitioners to make a firm distinction between the two conditions until the later nineteenth century.

Rickettsial and bacterial pathways

Typhus is a rickettsial infection which thrives in conditions of acute social dislocation, poverty and overcrowding and is principally, though not exclusively, encountered during the cold months of the year.[7] *Rickettsia prowazeki*, the infectious organism, which was first isolated in 1909, is transmitted from person to person by the body louse. The *rickettsiae* are ingested when the louse draws in blood from an individual already suffering from typhus; then, when this blood meal has been digested, the microorganisms are ejected with the faeces. In crowded and dirty living conditions, where lice and fleas proliferate, surface lesions, caused either by the bite of an insect or by the scratching of a persistent irritation, are inevitably common; and typhus is most usually spread when the *rickettsiae* contained in the faeces of lice are rubbed into broken skin. Once the disease has been contracted, the sufferer is afflicted by a severe headache and a very high temperature; and the entire body, except for the face, the palms of the hands and the soles of the feet, becomes rapidly disfigured by angry red spots. During an intense epidemic the case fatality rate may rise to more than 50 per cent; but during the nineteenth century it probably ranged between about 20 and 45 per cent.[8]

Unlike typhus, typhoid is a disease of the faecal-oral route, and is usually spread via infected water, milk and food.[9] There is no vector and transmission is always due either to passage from an already infected individual or from a carrier of the disease. Typhoid flourishes in all those circumstances in which the faeces of sufferers or immune carriers come into contact with extensively distributed supplies of food and drink. In contrast to typhus, typhoid has traditionally affected a wide range of both the poor and relatively affluent, particularly in societies in which water and foodstuffs have been exempt from effective public health regulations. Once the infection has been contracted, the patient becomes listless, loses appetite and then develops a high and sustained fever, which is often accompanied by profuse diarrhoea. This diarrhoea, leading to abdominal haemorrhage, is the most frequent terminal event in the illness. Typhoid, during the nineteenth century, was most common during the summer and autumn and case fatality was lower than that for typhus, fluctuating between about 15 and 20 per cent.[10]

The typhoid sufferer, like the individual who has contracted typhus, is liable to display a red rash, although its nature and distribution are, in fact, quite distinct. It was this symptom which persuaded most doctors before the later nineteenth century that the two conditions were identical. However, from the 1830s, a number of pioneers, notably W. W. Gerhard in America, P. C. A. Louis in Paris and Sir William Jenner in London, had drawn attention to prominent clinical differences between the two diseases, and especially to the fact that diarrhoea was never encountered in typhus.[11] Yet it was only in 1869 that William Farr at the Registrar-General's Office felt that it had become possible to collect separate national statistics for the *Annual Reports*. This failure to differentiate between the diseases makes it necessary to examine mortality attributable to them in two periods, before and after 1870. Mortality from typhus and typhoid, during the first period, was recorded as typhus; during the second, it was registered under typhus, typhoid and, a third category – simple continued fever. By the end of the first period typhus had gone into a steep decline as a cause of death and, during the second, it was replaced by typhoid as the most prevalent of the adult 'fevers' in

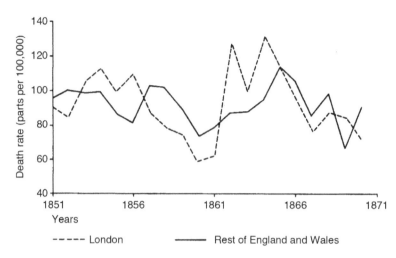

Figure 3.1   Mortality rate (parts per 100,000) from typhus and typhoid, London and the rest of England and Wales, 1851–70
Source: *Annual* and *Decennial Reports* of the Registrar-General

nineteenth-century Britain. Simple continued fever was of only limited statistical importance for a single transitional decade, the 1870s. In addition, there is strong evidence in favour of redistributing the mortality attributable to it to typhoid – a convention which has been followed in this chapter.[12]

Combined mortality from typhus and typhoid in London between 1851 and 1870 is plotted with mortality for the rest of England and Wales in Figure 3.1. Although it is not possible to make a definitive separation between the two infections during this first period, data from the London Fever Hospital, the only institution which accepted large numbers of working class fever patients before the 1870s, together with the observations of several medical officers of health, suggest that typhus probably accounted for a substantially higher proportion of mortality from the two diseases during the 1860s than the 1850s.[13]

This pattern is clearly revealed in Figure 3.2 which analyses the type of fever recorded for about 18,000 patients admitted to the London Fever Hospital between 1851 and 1870. Only once in the 1850s, during the recession associated with the end of the Crimean War in 1855–6, did contemporaries record that London had been

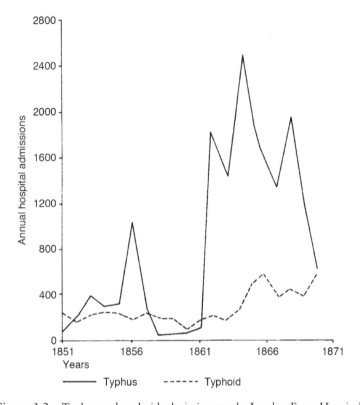

Figure 3.2   Typhus and typhoid admissions to the London Fever Hospital, 1851–70
Source: Charles Murchison, *The Continued Fevers of Great Britain* (London, 1884, 3rd edn), 52–3

afflicted by epidemic typhus.[14] However, from 1862 until 1870, the disease returned with unexpected ferocity and in 1869 and 1870 it was accompanied by an epidemic of the less fatal, jaundice-like infection, relapsing fever – popularly and aptly known as 'famine fever'.[15]

Throughout this period typhoid was an endemic or sub-epidemic rather than a consistently epidemic infection. Intermittently, though, during the 1850s, it may have accounted for as high an annual death toll as typhus. These peaks are probably inadequately documented in the London Fever Hospital records, since typhoid was a less visibly traumatic disease than typhus and a smaller proportion of total sufferers were admitted to hospital.[16] In particular, middle-class victims were unlikely to be accurately represented in public hospital records since they were reluctant to enter any institution such as the London Fever Hospital, which was partially reliant upon charitable funds.

Nevertheless, the testimony of several medical officers of health, from a wide geographical area within the capital, implies that intermittently during the 1850s, annual aggregate mortality from typhoid may have been greater than that from typhus.[17] District and hospital statistics, during the 1860s, gave the impression that mortality from the disease rose above its typically endemic norm to reach sub-epidemic proportions. The data from the London Fever Hospital indicate that between 1863 and 1870 deaths from typhoid followed the upward movement of typhus, although at lower absolute levels. The reduction in mortality from typhoid during the second period requires only brief description, following the decline of epidemic typhus from about 1870. Figure 3.3 shows the pattern for the capital, set against that for the rest of England and Wales.

The decline between 1871 and 1885, despite fluctuations, was both substantial and continuous. However, from 1885 until the end

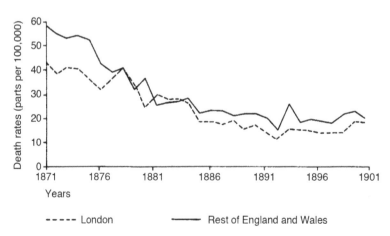

Figure 3.3 Mortality rate (parts per 100,000) from typhoid in London and the rest of England and Wales, 1871–1900
Source: *Annual* and *Decennial Reports* of the Registrar-General

of the century the rate of improvement slackened and little further progress was made either in the capital or in the rest of the country during the 1890s.[18]

It was after 1900 that mortality was rapidly and uninterruptedly reduced to levels which, by 1910, were beginning to approximate to the more sanguine expectations of the mid-twentieth century. A more detailed representation of mortality from the two diseases in London between 1851 and 1870 is set out in Table 3.1 and Figure 3.4. Since typhoid accounted for a higher proportion of aggregate mortality from the two infections between 1851 and 1860 than between 1861 and 1870, Figure 3.4 almost certainly under-estimates deaths from typhus during the 1860s. Thus, during the 1850s, only Shoreditch and Whitechapel experienced a combined death rate from typhus and typhoid of more than 110 per 100,000 population.

Yet, between 1861 and 1870 no East End district was exempt from very serious epidemic mortality from the two diseases, with typhus quite definitely claiming the bulk of the deaths.[19] The most telling illustration of this deterioration is provided by Poplar. In the earlier period its combined death rate from the two diseases was relatively low, comparable to that of such relatively affluent western and south western districts as Kensington, Marylebone and Wandsworth. However, as during the 1860s, the western, north western and south western suburbs marginally improved their position; Poplar, like the rest of the East End, was severely afflicted by epidemic typhus.

The decline in mortality from typhoid between 1870 and 1900 is shown in Table 3.1. The differentials in mortality between the poorest and the more affluent districts were now far less pronounced, especially after 1880, than had been the case for typhus during the preceding 20 years. In fact, by the beginning of the twentieth century, typhoid had ceased to be a major epidemic infection in the capital. A poor district in the East End, like Shoreditch, which had been particularly ravaged by both diseases during the 1850s and 1860s, had, by the 1890s, become very nearly totally immune from typhus and now only occasionally experienced annual death rates from typhoid of more than 15 per 100,000 population.

Table 3.1 Mortality from typhus and typhoid in London registration districts, 1851–1900 (death rates in parts per 100,000)

Districts	Typhus and typhoid		Typhoid 1871–80	Typhus 1871–80	Typhoid 1881–90	Typhoid 1891–1900
	1851–60	1861–70				
Kensington	61	54	21	5	22	10
Chelsea	77	70	29	6	16	13
Westminster*	87	81	32	6	23	27
Marylebone	68	61	27	4	18	13
Hampstead	65	31	20	–	19	11
Pancras	72	67	29	4	23	16
Islington	77	76	32	6	24	13
Hackney	83	71	33	7	27	13
St Giles	93	100	23	3	19	13
Holborn	78	100	30	6	19	16
City	104	136	48	7	29	18
Shoreditch	132	120	34	7	20	16
Bethnal Green	102	119	36	8	21	19
Whitechapel	116	135	42	6	30	13
St George in the East	100	152	35	10	17	17
Stepney and Mile End	101	123	32	8+	25	18
Poplar	70	113	32	5	24	19

(continued)

Table 3.1. (*continued*)

Districts	Typhus and typhoid		Typhoid 1871–80	Typhus 1871–80	Typhoid 1881–90	Typhoid 1891–1900
	1851–60	1861–70				
St Saviour**	92	98	32	6	15	17
St Olave[×]	103	101	34	7	20	17
Lambeth	76	85	35	7	25	12
Wandsworth	66	60	27	5	16	12
Camberwell	56	64	32	3	15	10
Greenwich	91	104	41	5	30	20
Lewisham	57	56	25	3	12	8
Woolwich	–	–	34	7⁺	12	4
London	87	89	30	5	18	12

Notes: *includes St George Hanover Square, Westminster; St Martin's, Westminster; St James and Strand districts

** includes St Saviour, St George and Newington

[×] includes St Olave, Bermondsey and Rotherhithe

⁺ doubtful value

Sources: Registrar-General, *Annual Reports* and *Supplements* to *Annual Reports*

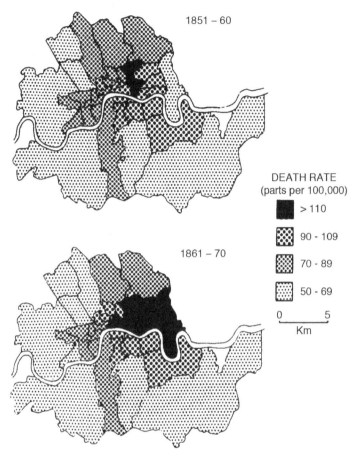

Figure 3.4   Mortality rate (parts per 100,000) from typhus and typhoid, London registration districts, 1851–60 and 1861–70
Source: *Annual* and *Decennial Reports* of the Registrar-General

Eras of decline: typhus

The decline of typhus has usually been explained in terms of an interraction between rising standards of living and the impact of the sanitary revolution – a long-established and inexplicit term covering large-scale improvements in drainage, water supply and housing, and associated levels of personal hygiene. When seeking to account for the decline of the disease after 1870, different historians have emphasized different variables subsumed under this generalized concept. Thus Creighton argued that an improved housing stock and greater communal attention to cleanliness had probably been less important than an increasingly healthy diet.[20]

George Rosen gave primacy to increased supplies of water which, so he contended, allowed more regular washing of both bodies and under-garments.[21] In the most rigorous analysis so far undertaken, Thomas McKeown and his colleagues have drawn attention to three related components: the direct effects of the systematic cleansing of the urban environment, improvements in diet, and the possibility of a favourable change in the relationship between host and parasite.[22] The emergence of a convincing and comprehensive account of the decline of typhus has clearly been inhibited by a number of conceptual and empirical difficulties. Therefore, in this section, existing, and often overlapping, explanations of the national reduction in mortality from the disease will be surveyed in the light of developments in the capital between about 1870 and 1900.

Whether as a means of cleansing the individual home, removing filth from enclosed streets and alleys, or raising levels of personal hygiene, an improved water supply has invariably occupied an important role within the traditional schema. In London, demographic pressure ensured that daily *per capita* supply declined marginally between the 1820s and 1850.[23] Consumption rose from 21 to 23 gallons per head per day during the 1850s, but the next 20 years witnessed little improvement and the water companies were under strong and persistent pressure to extend constant supply and to increase the meagre amounts delivered to the poorer areas for domestic purposes. By 1880 there had been an improvement, with *per capita* consumption within the capital as a whole rising to about 26 gallons per day.[24] If increases on this scale could be identified in those working class districts which had been most heavily affected by typhus during the 1860s, it might be possible to argue that this amelioration had played an important part in reducing the incidence of the disease in the 1870s. Yet detailed analysis of the evidence cannot support such a conclusion. The great bulk of the water consumed in the eastern and northern districts was supplied by the

New River and East London companies and, since these two concerns 'shared' many areas, statistics for aggregate supply from each company to individual registration districts are not available. However, a moderately reliable estimate of water consumption in the typhus-prone region as a whole – the eastern, inner city, inner northern and north eastern suburban districts shown in Figure 3.4 – can be calculated.

Per capita consumption in these districts rose from approximately 20 gallons per day in 1850 to 24 gallons by the mid-1870s.[25] This finding must, however, be set against the fact that it was only in the 1890s that more than 50 per cent of the total population in this region gained permanent access to company-supplied water and that, even at this late juncture, 31 per cent of all Londoners, and as many as 55 per cent of all customers of the New River Company, were still without constant supply.[26] It would clearly be rash, in the light of such statistics, to postulate a widespread change in working class washing habits, whether of bodies or of clothes, until a decade or so after typhus had entered its final decline.

Emphasis has also traditionally been placed on improved drainage. The period of intensive construction of sewers in the capital, both by district and municipal authorities, beginning with the Chadwickian initiative in the late 1840s, and culminating in the completion of the main drainage project in the mid-1860s, undoubtedly witnessed the transportation of very large quantities of refuse from closed inner city areas to the larger external environment.[27] Yet in the absence, until the mid-1860s, of an efficient means of extra-urban sewage disposal, or even moderately reliable methods of water treatment, any reduction in mortality from typhus which may have flowed from less insalubrious living conditions in the inner city, was almost certainly cancelled out by an increase in mortality attributable to water-transmitted infections. This hypothesis is supported not only by the rising share of deaths from typhoid within combined mortality from typhus and typhoid but also by the timing and intensity of the water-transmitted cholera epidemics which afflicted the capital in 1848–9, 1854–5 and 1866.[28] According to this interpretation, the systematic drainage of the inner city districts which was undertaken during the sanitary revolution may indeed have reduced mortality from typhus but only at the short-term cost of a deterioration in water supplies drawn from river sources which were still too close to major sewer outlets.[29] Once the main drainage system had been completed in the mid-1860s, London certainly became a cleaner and a healthier place in which to live and, in this sense, there can be little doubt that improved sewerage was a necessary, though not a sufficient, condition for the eradication of epidemic typhus.

The next strand in the traditional argument concerns the provision of housing and on this issue the metropolitan evidence may be briefly and categorically summarized. Neither contemporary medical specialists, nor urban historians, have been able to point to any significant reduction in overcrowding until about 20 years after typhus had ceased to be an epidemic threat.[30] The possible impact of an improved diet is a complicated issue. The East End suffered extreme poverty, involving malnutrition and even occasional cases of starvation, during the extended typhus epidemic of the 1860s.[31] In the light of trends now generally accepted for the country as a whole, it seems unlikely that standards of living failed to rise marginally when typhus waned for the last time in these same areas during the 1870s.[32] Twentieth century epidemiologists and medical historians are undecided, however, as to the relationship between fluctuations in nutrition and changes in communal resistance to typhus, especially when nutrition is isolated from the generalized nexus of poverty, overcrowding and vagrancy in which the disease was observed to flourish in the nineteenth century.[33] It is certainly unwise to seek links, however tentative, between, for example, the price of bread and the incidence of typhus in the capital during the 1850s and 1860s.[34]

The evident shortcomings of the argument that either the impact of the sanitary revolution, or rising standards of living, can adequately account for the sudden and dramatic decline in mortality from typhus after about 1870 are thrown into even sharper relief when the metropolitan statistics between 1851 and 1880 are set against those for other large centres of population in England and

Table 3.2   Mortality from typhus and typhoid in selected towns, 1851–80 (death rates in parts per 100,000)

Major towns	1851–60	1861–70	Percentage change	1871–80	Approximate percentage change
Belfast	–	123*	–	91	−26
Birmingham	107	79	−26	2	−97
Blackburn	157	110	−30	I	−98
Bolton	107	95	−7	2	−98
Bradford	98	106	+8	5	−95
Brighton	91	53	−42	–	−96
Bristol	99	93	−6	3	−98
Dublin	–	130*	–	96	−26
Hull	124	144	+16	1	−99
Leeds	109	141	+29	11	−92
Leicester	137	80	−42	1	−99
Liverpool	154	222	+44	58	−73
London	87	89	+2	5	−94
Manchester	124	170	+37	18	−78
Newcastle	99	128	+29	14	−78
Nottingham	105	85	−19	2	−98
Norwich	104	90	−13	–	−98
Oldham	90	85	−5	–	−98
Preston	109	84	−23	–	−98
Salford	83	135	+63	1	−97
Sheffield	132	139	+5	8	−88
Stoke	92	97	+5	–	−96
Sunderland	80	92	+15	33	−64

Note: *1864–75

Source: Registrar-General, *Annual Reports* and *Supplements* to *Annual Reports*; Registrar-General for Ireland, *Annual Reports* and *Supplements* to *Annual Reports*

Ireland.[35] Table 3.2 seeks to compare mortality rates from typhus, as well as changes in those rates, in 22 conurbations of more than 100,000 population at the census of 1881. Since the figures for 1851–60 and 1861–70 refer to typhus and typhoid combined, and those for 1871–80 to typhus alone, there is clearly a lack of comparability between the second and fourth columns. Yet, even if the conservative estimate is made that as few as 50 per cent of all deaths from typhus and typhoid in the 1860s were in fact attributable to typhus, only two communities – Belfast and Dublin – reveal an annual average reduction of less than the remarkably high figure of 60 per cent during the 1870s. This is a decline sufficiently large, sudden and generalized throughout the majority of urban areas, to hypothesize that it may have been an 'autonomous' change in the nature of the disease itself, rather than numerous uncoordinated programmes of reform, directed at differing environments, which precipitated the once-and-for-all extinction of epidemic typhus in nineteenth-century England. When, however, the case-fatality rate for the disease during the early nineteenth century, when aggregate mortality was high, is compared with case fatality during the later decades of the century, when mortality had been so greatly diminished, the result – a rate consistently fluctuating between about 20 and 45 per cent – does not indicate that the infective *rickettsiae* were becoming less virulent.

There is, in other words, no evidence to support the view that *rickettsia prowazeki* was undergoing a modification during the later nineteenth century similar to that proposed by McKeown and Record for the haemolytic streptoccocus responsible for the propagation of scarlet fever.[36] Epidemic typhus was certainly becoming rarer after 1870, but the chances of survival for the individual who contracted it, during the 1890s, for example, were no higher than they had been for his or her predecessors at mid-century.[37] Nevertheless, what of the vector? Is it conceivable that there may have been a sudden diminution in the body louse population, or a favourable shift in the relationship between body louse and *rickettsia*, which resulted either in fewer lice coming into contact with susceptible humans, or the same number of lice transmitting *rickettsiae*, though to less destructive effect?[38] Unfortunately, it is not possible to locate evidence which would either support definitively or contradict the hypothesis that the relationship between the body louse and *rickettsia prowazeki* did undergo a modification of this kind; but the stability of the case-fatality rate among human sufferers from typhus makes it improbable

that such an ecological event did occur. Yet there is a case for
proposing that, from the early 1870s, the great English
conurbations were becoming increasingly insulated from foci of
infection and, hence, also from regions in which there were high
concentrations of body lice – notably in urban Ireland (Table 3.2).
The final column of Table 3.2 demonstrates that typhus continued to
thrive in Dublin and Belfast, and that among English urban areas
the disease was declining less rapidly in those trading and seaborne
centres in the north- east and the north-west which had natural and
continuing links with Ireland.[39] The wider context within which
this 'lagged' effect should be located is one in which, taking England
and Wales as a whole, the number of Irish-born residents had risen
very rapidly from approximately 300,000 in 1841 to just over
600,000 in 1861, but had then remained static for the next four
decades at around half a million.[40]

In London, the Irish-born accounted for nearly 5 per cent of the
total population in 1851, just under 4 per cent in 1861, 2.1 per cent
in 1881 and 1.6 per cent in 1891.[41] It would clearly be a caricature
of social and epidemiological history to use these figures to argue
that successive waves of epidemic typhus in nineteenth-century
Britain were determined by the 'flow of infection' from Ireland, or
that the decline of the disease coincided symmetrically and causally
with diminishing immigration after 1860. Nevertheless, once it
had run its full epidemic course, the extended and final outbreak of
typhus could be reactivated only by a large-scale movement of
infected lice-carrying individuals from centres of population where
there continued to be a high incidence of the disease. Such centres
were to be found in Dublin and Belfast at precisely that time when,
had it conformed to the general periodicity observable during
the first 80 years of the century, the disease would have been
expected to recur in the great English cities. However, this time,
typhus did not return. This remission is more likely to be
understood by an analysis of short-term fluctuations in rates of
migration from Ireland to urban England than through a
generalized appeal to a supposedly monolithic and nationally
uniform sanitary revolution.

Eras of decline: typhoid

The decline of typhoid during the final 30 years of the nineteenth century may be more briefly considered. Despite incompatibilities between the measures undertaken to reduce mortality and the theories which supported them, the conscious efforts of doctors and professional epidemiologists played a more significant role in this process than had been the case with typhus. Throughout this period epidemiology continued to be shaped by a broadly miasmatic theory of disease, according to which small-scale outbreaks of typhoid were believed to be transmitted via the vapours which emanated from badly constructed privies and water closets.[42] The programmes which were undertaken as the practical expression of these beliefs undoubtedly reduced much mortality which would now be attributed to person-to-person infection. There was, therefore, no functional contradiction between a predominantly miasmatic conception and the emergent and more 'scientific' approach which emphasized the specificity of the disease.

From about 1870, improvements in company filtration techniques ensured that unsafe water ceased to be widely suspected by public health workers and, subsequently, attention was directed towards other ways in which the disease was believed to be spread. Unsafe milk and foodstuffs were energetically tracked down in the 1870s and 1880s;[43] contaminated shellfish and water-cress were frequently implicated in the 1890s;[44] and, by the end of the century, investigators were beginning to understand the role of the immune carrier.[45] Attention was briefly redirected in the 1890s to puzzling differentials in district mortality rates from typhoid. The possibility that the disease had once again been transmitted via public water supplies was widely canvassed. Shirley Forster Murphy, the first medical officer of health to the London County Council, pointed to the probability that districts which were supplied from the Lea were likely to suffer higher mortality than those supplied from the Thames and, more specifically, that the reservoirs and filters of the East London and New River Companies were inadequate to the task of providing safe water when the Lea was in flood.[46]

Murphy's methodology was sophisticated and revealing. He demonstrated, by applying Booth's data on poverty to the incidence of infectious disease for each of the metropolitan districts, that in the case of typhoid, and typhoid only, complex environmental shortcomings were more significant than differentials in real income.[47] This was a telling formulation of several of the aetiological differences which had long been thought to exist between typhoid and typhus, as well as an explanation of the frequently observed phenomenon whereby typhoid had invaded even the most respectable and hygienically scrupulous of middle-class homes.[48]

In addition, by the 1890s compulsory notification and hospitalization in public institutions administered by the Metropolitan Asylums Board had been added to routine inspection and epidemiological analysis at district level. Thirty per cent of all metropolitan typhoid sufferers, by the end of the decade, were receiving treatment as in-patients.[49] The geographical spread, and mortality from outbreaks of the disease were reduced by this extension of hospital provision to that section of the working class just above that officially stigmatized as 'pauperized'.[50] Thus the London experience suggests that McKeown and Record's generally pessimistic conclusions *vis-à-vis* the impact of hospitalization on infectious disease during the nineteenth century as a whole may be in need of modification.[51] It is worth noting that, by the end of the century, the public fever hospitals had been augmented by local bacteriological laboratories which facilitated a more rapid identification of localized outbreaks.[52]

The steady elimination of typhoid during the final 30 years of the century proceeded despite, rather than because of, the initiative of any unifying municipal body with responsibility for the whole of London. The powers of the Metropolitan Board of Works had been deliberately restricted in this sphere by the Act of 1855 and, after 1889, the medical officer of health to the London County Council occupied no more than an advisory position in relation to the still intensely independent and localist vestries. A closer and more effective control over the environment may be traced to the enthusiastic involvement of a network of specialists who came into contact with one another through a variety of professional and scientific bodies which had their headquarters in the capital. The water supply improved consistently, with only intermittent set-backs, between 1870 and the formation of the Metropolitan Water Board in 1902.

This improvement occurred not through government surveillance exercised by the Board of Trade, but as a result of the collaboration between William Farr at the Registrar-General's Office and the eminent theoretical chemist and water analyst, Edward Frankland – a relationship which began during the cholera crisis of 1866 and which survived, in the face of acrimonious opposition from the water companies, for the next 15 years.[53] Frankland may well have exaggerated the dangers of the Thames and the Lea as long-term sources of supply,[54] but without his regular reports on chemical and bacteriological quality, stringent and quasi-compulsory metropolitan water standards would not have been adopted. Once the safety of the water supply had been finally and compulsorily ensured, mortality from typhoid could be eroded by other means. The Metropolitan Association of Medical Officers of Health, reporting on specific epidemics, pressing for more rigorous protection of food and milk, and rebuking recalcitrant vestries, complemented and extended the efforts of Frankland and Farr.[55] The influence of these individuals, operating within a still largely informal administrative network, and undertaking regular measures to control not only typhoid, but the whole spectrum of infectious diseases, should not be underestimated.[56]

Typhoid, therefore, seems to have been brought at least partially under control by the campaign launched against it by doctors, epidemiologists and public health workers, while typhus, a more complex, socially traumatic and threatening disease, was less tractable. The two infections, frequently and understandably confused by contemporaries, and later unhelpfully bracketed together as 'dirt diseases' by historians of public health, reacted quite differently to attempts at coordinated containment. At the explicit level this chapter has attempted to confront some of the ambiguities and contradictions of the orthodox, 'classic' sanitary revolution; implicitly, it has touched upon a deeper and more enduring problem – the troubled issue of agency in history.

A note on sources

In all but the last of the *Supplements* to the *Annual Reports* which apply to the period under discussion, the Registrar-General claimed that deaths in public institutions, including hospitals, had been redistributed to the 'normal district of residence'. However, a readjustment of this kind was never undertaken for district death-rates from specific causes. The tables and maps in this chapter, therefore, have attempted to reduce serious misrepresentation by modifying the Registrar-General's statistics in the light of data available from those hospitals which admitted large numbers of fever patients. The following points should be noted.

1851–70: Deaths occurring in the London Fever Hospital, which was situated in Islington, have been reallocated to district of residence, following the extensive admissions data contained in Charles Murchison, *A Treatise on the Continued Fevers of Great Britain* (London, 1884), 74–5. Third edition, edited by W. Cayley.

1871–90: Some distortion was caused by the admission of growing numbers of fever patients to hospitals administered by the Metropolitan Asylums Board in Hackney, Lambeth and Greenwich. Adjustment has been made by applying approximate case fatality rates to data contained in the regular listings of case admissions to the various hospitals in the *Minutes* of the Metropolitan Asylums Board for each of the relevant years: and for 1887–90, in *Annual Reports* of the Statistical Committee of the Metropolitan Asylums Board.

1891–1900: Because of the dramatic increase in hospitalization in this period, many of the Registrar-General's figures for mortality at district level are quite meaningless. It is, however, fortunate that cases of infectious disease at district level began to be recorded annually from 1890 onwards. These statistics constitute probably the most comprehensive source for disease incidence for any late nineteenth-century city, and they may be located in the pull-out tables and graphs attached to the *Annual Reports* of the Statistical Committee of the Metropolitan Asylums Board, 1890–1902.[57]

CHAPTER 4

THE FINAL CATASTROPHE: CHOLERA IN LONDON, 1866

Calamity on epidemic calamity

In 1866 pandemic cholera attacked Britain for the fourth and final time in an epidemic which struck with extreme ferocity in the East End of London, killing very nearly 4,000 people there between the end of July and the beginning of November.[1] The epidemic has not yet received attention either from social historians or in the literature of the history of medicine. It is, however, generally agreed in each of the existing accounts that it was the action (or, rather the negligent inaction) of the East London Water Company which decisively determined the dissemination and scale of the outbreak.[2] An analysis of time structure and localized patterns of mortality reinforces such an interpretation.[3]

The intention of this chapter, then, is not in any sense revisionist, for posthumous exoneration cannot be proffered where it is so evidently undeserved. It seeks rather to illuminate the extraordinarily diverse spectrum of attitudes towards water-transmitted disease which were in competition for intellectual and social hegemony in Britain and shows that it was only a minority within what may be loosely characterized as the nascent *avant garde* of epidemiology which gave unqualified support to the view that the outbreak of 1866 was decisively carried by water. Any total account must separate out a multiplicity of epidemiological and socio-medical theories as a complement to the incontestable conclusion, which may be – and indeed was – deduced from the statistics of district mortality collected by William Farr at the Registrar-General's Office, that the epidemic was primarily spread by unsafe water. But to the great majority of those who specialized in medicine and the protection of public health in the 1860s such a supposition smacked of scientific error and social irresponsibility.

The chapter falls into four parts. The first is a brief chronological outline of the epidemic, described principally and deliberately from the perspective of two progressives – William Farr and Edward Frankland – who were directly involved in monitoring mortality and possible modes of transmission. In the second, the company's defensive strategy is situated within the mainstream of consensus medical ideology, exemplified here by the writings and public statements of the metropolitan medical officers of health. There is then an analysis of the findings of the various parliamentary and departmental investigations which, either directly or indirectly, set themselves the task of evaluating the precise degree of culpability of the East London Company. Finally, attention is given to the orientation and testimony of those influential statesmen of the new medical science – notably John Simon and John Netten Radcliffe – who were strategically placed to modify future systems of administrative control and public health legislation.

By the end of July 1866, mortality in the East End had reached traumatic levels and William Farr at the Registrar-General's Office was already well aware of the probable role of unsafe water in the transmission of the epidemic. He was also pessimistic about the possibilities of preventative action. 'The Company will no doubt take exemplary pains to filter its water', he told his confidant and informal scientific adviser, Edward Frankland, 'but it is not easy to guarantee the purity of water drawn from such a river as the Lea, in dangerous proximity to sewers, cuts and canals'.[4] On July 30 in another letter to Frankland, he reiterated his contention that there must be a connection between the abnormal contamination of the Lea and the

spiraling death-rate in the East End and, on the following day, he
was telling Frankland that the epidemic 'quite reminds me of the
Southwark slaughter' of a dozen years earlier.[5] Some kind of rapid
action was imperative but, when approached informally, the East
London Company bridled at the suggestion that it might be even
minimally responsible for the dissemination of the disease: and on
August 2, in an attempt to stifle damaging rumours, Charles
Greaves, the company engineer, who was to play a dramatic role in
the subsequent unravelling of the tragedy, wrote to *The Times* giving
an assurance that the water which was being drawn from the Lea was
absolutely safe.[6] This was in partial response to Farr's statement that
use was still being made of a canal which connected the company's
filter beds at one of their works directly with the river.

Unknown to Greaves, Farr had already examined detailed maps
and, to his intense indignation, had discovered that there were in fact
two pumping establishments – at Old Ford and at Lea Bridge. At the
former, besides a covered reservoir, there were also two others which
were not covered. Whatever the exact means of transmission of
cholera in the East End, therefore, the company had clearly
contravened a clause of the Metropolitan Water Act of 1852 which
outlawed uncovered reservoirs within five miles of St Paul's.[7]

Greaves's response was forthright. He accused the Registrar's
Office of consulting out-of-date maps and went on to insist that,
although the canal had yet to be filled in, '... not a drop of unfiltered
water has for several years past been supplied by the company for any
purpose'.[8] But the existence of the uncovered reservoir had already
temporarily undermined the company's position and Farr now moved
swiftly. On August 3 he wrote to Frankland's assistant: 'The engineer,
Mr. Greaves, states that there is still a connection between the *wells* of
the engines at *Old Ford* and the uncovered reservoirs, but denies that
these waters are ever used.' To test the reliability of this assertion,
Farr asked the assistant to undertake rigorous analyses of water from
the single covered and from the two uncovered reservoirs at Old Ford,
as well as at the Lea Bridge works both before and after filtration.[9]
Predictably, the chemical analysis revealed nothing and the
repercussions which flowed from this unsuccessful effort to identify

the presence of the cholera 'poison' – the terminology legitimized by
John Snow and now freely deployed by the progressives – were to
prove of exceptional methodological significance in the controversy
which ensued.

Searching for hidden explanations

Both during and in the immediate aftermath of the virulent
epidemic, the company retaliated against the accusations of
'progressives' by citing authoritative miasmatic and sociological
theories of disease which purported to explain the peculiar
vulnerability of the poorest and least hygienic districts of the East
End. N. Beardmore, the engineer to the River Lea Trust, wrote to the
Registrar's Office on 6 August to insist that: '... overcrowding,
deficiency of drainage, and inferior articles of food are more likely to
have promoted cholera than impurity or deficiency of water'. The
East End, he went on, was populated by '... dock labourers, sailors,
mechanics in the new factores [sic], and great numbers of laundresses',
all social groups whose poverty, irregular lives and underdeveloped
sense of personal hygiene made them especially susceptible to the
disease.[10]

The company was also able to rely on the open or tacit support of a
majority of the metropolitan medical officers of health. The acting
officer for Mile End Old Town claimed that he had 'never seen or read
a single reliable fact' to support the water theory.[11] His colleagues
were less extreme but they nevertheless endorsed a wide range of
alternative hypotheses which implicitly minimized the direct
influence of unsafe water. Sociological schema of the kind that
Beardmore had championed, based on allegedly empirical
observations which emphasized poverty *per se*, the influence of social
class and a dissolute way of life, were held to be more persuasive than
the exclusive water theory. There was also a continuing commitment
to the atmospheric 'Thames-borne' theory of infection, first
propounded by William Farr in his then pioneering work on
elevation, meteorology and the 'epidemic atmosphere' in 1849 and
1854.[12] 'The present epidemic', explained the medical officer for

Greenwich, who was clearly attracted to this kind of theoretical framework, 'has mainly existed in all parts of my district as are contiguous to the River Thames. The nearer the river, the more cases of cholera, and the greater the severity of attacks generally, the disease gradually decreasing in virulence and numbers as the distance increases from the river.'[13]

But by far the most popular total explanation to which the medical officers subscribed was the well-tried generalized Chadwickian hierarchy of '... bad water, bad air, defective drainage, overcrowding, dirty and irregular habits', with the important proviso that it was invariably traditional non-specific miasmatic conditions, and not unsafe water *per se* which occupied a determining position.[14] By this period, the seemingly indefinitely flexible miasmatic doctrine had also incorporated elements of Pettenkofer's more rigorous soil theory of disease.[15] 'There certainly is a difference between the mortality of the parts supplied by the three water companies', the medical officer for Kensington recorded, 'but I do not attribute this at all to the water, but rather to the drainage, overcrowding, and more especially the clay soil of the northern part'.[16] It was Thomas Orton, medical officer to the Limehouse district, and a combative though fair and thorough opponent of the 'exclusive' water theory, who provided the most acute summary of the various explanations which were championed by activists in the public health movement in London in the mid-1860s.[17]

The validity of his assertion that '... pretty generally amongst all classes the theory of the water poison is repudiated... especially among the poor' is open to the objection that many ordinary people do seem to have been aware of at least some of the dangers of drinking unsafe water.[18] But his catalogue of favoured hypotheses on the causation of cholera – an even more richly variegated crop that had been canvassed and found wanting in 1849 and 1854 – was comprehensive and authoritative. Orton identified as many as a dozen epidemiological schools and splinter groups. A powerful section of the medical establishment continued to insist on the primacy of meteorological phenomena, but there was also influential advocacy of a more accurate observation both of telluric variables and subtle changes in the level of atmospheric ozone and electricity. Among the growing numbers of modern and scientific medical thinkers, who were conversant with the work of Liebig and Pasteur, Orton recorded support for the concept of zymotic fermentation, although there were serious divergences as to precisely which agent – fungus, animalicular body or poison – was alleged to underlay the disease process. The most significant aspect of the survey, however, was the relegation of the distinctive corpus of ideas explicitly associated with the names of Budd and Snow to the most comprehensively criticized and rejected of the poison-based categories.[19] Even when proper allowance has been made for Orton's own prejudices, here was potent confirmation of a profound animosity among public health workers both to the exclusive water theory and the emerging notion of the specificity of disease.[20]

It might be concluded from this analysis that the metropolitan medical officers of the mid-1860s had no interest in water quality: but such an assertion would be over-dogmatic. Given the existing, although, as we have seen, confused, consensus on the mechanism of spread of infectious disease, it was inevitable that it would be the issue of quantity rather than quality which would claim the greater attention. If houses and bodies could be kept clean, it was argued, the general death-rate would decline dramatically. But the companies' refusal to extend constant supply and their draconian policy towards poor tenants who fell behind with their payments, or who misunderstood or failed to comply with a by now complex body of regulations, retarded progress.[21] In a political and environmental context of this kind questions of quantity and quality became intertwined and inseparable. For where dwellings or even whole courts were dependent on either a common butt, or on an inadequately serviced cistern, what became known as domestic pollution was inevitable.[22]

The attraction to medical officers of this particular explanation of the process of infection was that it could be accommodated both within the generalized miasmatic doctrine as well as within a looser version of the exclusive water theory. According to the former, emanations from an unsafe cistern interacted with atmospheric impurities to produce disease: according to the latter, cholera or typhoid, in a sense which was never clearly defined, was quite simply swallowed. Thus it was that before, during and after the epidemic of 1866, medical officers sustained a powerful campaign for constant supply and regular cleansing of domestic storage systems.[23] This was a programme which could be advocated without violation of a total belief system still resistant to incorporation of the exclusive water theory.[24]

Defending the indefensible?

It was within the context of this diverse but not wholly hostile set of theories and counter-theories that the East London Company set about its defence. It was especially fortunate in being able to call upon the services of Henry Letheby, Simon's successor as medical officer to the City of London, who had regularly tested its water in his capacity as analyst to the Association of Medical Officers of Health.[25] Letheby, one of the most able critics of the water-borne theory, pointed to the technical and methodological difficulties of actually locating the inferred cholera poison.[26] He made telling use of the by now familiar argument that '... teetotallers and others who drank largely of the East London Water in its unboiled condition, ... had been signally exempt from the disease',[27] and that it would have been equally convincing (or unconvincing) to canvass the proposition that the epidemic had been transmitted by a common gas supply.[28] He dwelt at length on the implications of closed institutions where there had been heavy consumption of East London water but relatively low mortality, defying supporters of the exclusive theory to explain such an apparent anomaly.[29]

Letheby's eloquently destructive skills were badly needed, for by Christmas 1866 the company's case had been apparently fatally weakened by Charles Greaves's sudden and unabashed admission that there had indeed been what he described as an 'implied sanction' to draw upon unfiltered water during periods of exceptionally high demand.[30] It is an indication of the continuing novelty of the water theory that the only justification that Greaves felt impelled to submit was that Letheby had assured him that the unfiltered water which had been stored for emergency delivery was of the highest standard. And Frankland's assistant, in the emergency analysis which has already been noted, had not been able to dispute this judgement on chemical grounds. In the light of Greaves' confession, the formal report by the Board of Trade could not be anything but harsh, yet, from the company's point of view, it was not wholly condemnatory. 'A distinct infringement of the provisions of the 1852 Act' had indeed occurred, but the inspector was not prepared to grant the East End complainants their case in full.[31]

The crucial rider was phrased in the following terms: '... any poison so distributed would have been in a condition, if it were soluble in water, of considerable dilution; and I am not prepared on that account, as well as in consideration of other respects of their district, to go as far as the Memorialists, in asserting that this water was the principal if not the sole cause of the fearful mortality from cholera'.[32] In other reports concerned with the allocation of blame for the outbreak, this 'deplorable state' of the East End was made to carry a heavier burden: and what has been designated in this chapter as the sociological explanation tended to be given priority over any theory which isolated a specific infective medium.

Although the Rivers Pollution Commissioners deplored the company's laxness in distributing filtered supplies which had then been immediately subjected to admixture with untreated water, they also drew pointed attention to insanitary local conditions.[33] Similarly, the framers of the report of the Select Committee on East London Water Bills, which had originally been drafted in the immediate aftermath of the epidemic, noting an 'entire concurrence',[34] with the Board of Trade's castigation of the company under the Act of 1852, subsequently revised their conclusions as follows: 'We think it right to observe that the evidence leads to the opinion that the spread of cholera might equally be ascribed to defective sanitary arrangements and to other causes.'[35] In such a climate, the East London Company could counter-attack with a degree of confidence and, in July 1867, the directors wrote to the Board of Trade disputing the implications which had inevitably been drawn from the inspector's report by the public at large, and seeking what amounted to an official pardon.[36] Carefully pre-selected phrases which the inspector, for reasons of scientific accuracy, had allowed to stand in a deliberately tentative form,were taken from their context and skilfully presented to give the impression that the company had been misrepresented and unjustly maligned. The directors minimized the misdemeanours of 1866, while simultaneously congratulating themselves on undertaking improvements which were, so they claimed, neither required of them by law, nor by prevailing views on the prevention of infectious disease.[37]

The Board of Trade, however, declined to reconsider its verdict.[38] By late 1867 public and specialist opinion had hardened against the company's unrepentant arrogance. In the summer of 1866, William Farr had spoken with deliberate and measured ambiguity of this 'disastrous accident in East London'.[39] Now the invariably moderate *British Medical Journal*, which continued to support a broadly miasmatic theory of cholera transmission, presented evidence which revealed that on several occasions in 1864 and 1865 as well as in 1866, the company had delivered unfiltered water.[40] According to the more militant *Lancet*, the company had knowingly taken advantage of the scientific and technical difficulties surrounding the chemical identification of the postulated cholera poison.[41] Such critics had not suddenly been converted to the exclusive water theory: what they considered intolerable was that a company which had been given great power over the welfare of the capital, had not hesitated to break the law, while simultaneously arguing that the law itself was redundant.

Hunches and revolutionary theories

The most influential of the public health specialists, John Simon, now urged that the companies be finally subjected to more intensive and better informed public surveillance. 'The power of life and death', he declaimed, 'in commercial hands is something for which, till recently, there has been no precedent in the world, and even yet the public seems but slightly awake to its importance.' But

significantly, and like so many others, he went on to lament the
failure of existing techniques of chemical analysis to provide evidence
of the existence of the cholera 'poison'.[42] When he directly addressed
the scientific community, Simon was even more cautious in his
assessment of the causation of the epidemic. Netten Radcliffe had
prepared an outspoken critique of the behaviour of the East London
Company for the Medical Office of the Privy Council. In a
characteristically incisive addendum to Radcliffe's report, Simon
asked rhetorically: '. . . for the substance of Mr. Radcliffe's conclusion
is it necessary to assume that the water was drunk?' and then
proceeded to put the weight of his authority behind an account cast
in Pettenkofer's terminology.[43] Scrupulous scientist and symbolic
protector of public health that he was, Simon could not accept
hypotheses which had yet to be fully verified under laboratory
conditions or through irrefutable statistical and epidemiological
research: his strength, as Royston Lambert has noted, lay precisely in
his ability to reconcile the progressive and consensus views which
have been the subject of the journal.[44] Radcliffe, on the other hand,
seems to have been more aware of the urgent need to refute
miasmatically-based doctrine in order to dramatize the potential
dangers of water and river pollution, to rebuke the water companies,
and to weaken the appeal of what appeared to him to be an over-
exclusively sociological and hence non-scientific account of the mode
of transmission of infectious disease.

The two most convincing counter-arguments to the exclusive
theory, which we have seen stated by the articulate Henry Letheby,
were, first, that there was no known practical means of demonstrating
the existence of the cholera poison; and, second, that large numbers of
consumers of allegedly unsafe supplies had nevertheless escaped
infection. To neutralize the first objection Radcliffe drew upon the
voluminous data gathered during the country-wide statistical surveys
undertaken by Simon's department. If this body of evidence was
analysed objectively, he contended, then it was clear enough that
cholera and typhoid would not '. . . attain general prevalence in a
town except where the faulty water supply develops them'.[45] To the
second criticism, which postulated an alleged logical inconsistency as

much as any empirical flaw, he urged that '... the positive and generally more applicable facts may justly, and for practical purposes, warrant a conclusion apparently in contradiction with certain negative facts of much more restricted application'.[46] Logic, in other words, must be tempered by the dictates of commonsense: the reality of epidemiological fieldwork, warts and all, must replace the caricature so readily derided by armchair sanitarians.

But Radcliffe was expressing a minority view even within the untypical set of beliefs shared by the vanguard of the public health movement: of the major figures involved, only Farr and Frankland could be counted as unequivocal allies. In the absence of tests for specificity, of a generally agreed *modus operandi* for the inferred cholera poison, as well as an only primitive knowledge of the precise bacteriological effects of filtration on raw river water, what might seem to have been the deliberately deceitful obduracy of the East London Company and its apologists, may be more meaningfully located within its proper historical context. Nor need this be interpreted as exoneration for, as we have already noted, the directors and the engineer had indeed flouted the law, and later, tortuously attempted to justify actions which the law condemned. It is, however, necessary to be clear about both the nature and the aims of the Metropolitan Water Act of 1852, as well as of popular attitudes to water-transmitted disease in the mid-1860s. It is tempting to assume that the provisions which outlawed the use of water from uncovered reservoirs and which insisted on 'adequate' filtration were devised rigorously and specifically to prevent large-scale epidemics of the most dangerous water-transmitted diseases, cholera and typhoid. But such an assumption cannot be sustained. The mid-century debate over water supply in London centred more on matters of political and economic control than the effects of unsafe water on public health;[47] and the conservative stance of the medical officers of health a dozen years later demonstrated a continuing scepticism to the radical ideas which had first been proposed by John Snow and William Budd.[48]

Despite Thomas Orton's confident generalizations to the contrary, broad associations between unsafe and unfiltered water and bad health were widely accepted among the population at large. But causal connections were only rarely made explicit and were more likely to be intuited by ordinary people than embraced by specialists in social medicine. In this sense, the East Londoner who found a dead and decomposing eel in his supply pipe in 1866 and moved immediately to the conclusion that the East London Company had been responsible for the dissemination of cholera, was closer to a correct analysis than the miasmatist who tended to propound the more generalized sociological schema which has been discussed in this chapter.[49]

During the next 25 years, the miasmatic paradigm was finally supplanted by the emerging concept of a still largely inferred germ theory of disease, but the effects of this change on epidemiological and public health practice were by no means pre-ordained. William Farr's long-standing ideal had been a predictive theory which would rest, rock-like, on an accumulated body of statistical observation;[50] but for obvious practical and theoretical reasons, this was no more likely to be attained in 1866 than it was a hundred years later. Another school of practitioners, directly descended from the miasmatists, remained loyal to Pettenkofer's postulates which implicitly minimized the possibility of laying bare exact correlations between mortality and any single, given environmental variable. In the long run, however, it was Netten Radcliffe's persuasively commonsensical although almost excessively non-doctrinaire advocacy of the detailed analysis of each epidemic within the parameters of a tested corpus of mutually reinforcing medical, scientific and epidemiological knowledge, which eventually superseded its rivals. According to this approach, it was imperative to act *as though* unsafe water was likely to have been the primary medium during any wide-ranging outbreak of cholera or typhoid, and in the 30 years following the epidemic of 1866 it provided the ground-rules for an increasingly efficient surveillance of the metropolitan water supply.[51]

This chapter has discussed a single event – the traumatic cholera epidemic which afflicted the East End of London in 1866 – in an attempt to cast light on a more general historical topic: the extent to which laymen and specialists in public health during the 1860s accepted or rejected the theory that infectious disease might be decisively transmitted by unsafe water. It has been suggested that it was only an elite within an elite – notably William Farr, Edward Frankland and Netten Radcliffe – that was willing to subscribe whole-heartedly to the view that the cholera had been spread *via* unsafe water, distributed by the East London Water Company. Other progressive thinkers, and, most significantly, John Simon, chose to assess the epidemic in terms that were still heavily influenced by classical miasmatic doctrine; and a majority of the medical officers of health lent their authority to interpretations which reinforced the water company's contention that no single version of the emerging germ theory of disease could adequately explain the course of the outbreak.

In the longer term, the water company's ill-fated admission that it had knowingly flouted the provisions of the Metropolitan Water Act of 1852 provoked widespread public hostility; and, in the aftermath of the epidemic, it was this miscalculation, rather than any transformation in popular attitudes towards the role of water in the spread of disease, which triggered demands for more rigorous public control of the water companies. The 'final catastrophe' of 1866 – and, especially, Edward Frankland and Netten Radcliffe's consistently outspoken and unambiguous indictment of the 'water poison' – had a decisive impact on water treatment policies during the final 30 years of the nineteenth century.

CHAPTER 5

THE METROPOLITAN AND THE MUNICIPAL: THE POLITICS OF HEALTH AND ENVIRONMENT, 1860-1920

Dimensions of governmental 'amateurism'

As David Reeder pointed out in a major historiographical survey in the early 1980s, many contemporaries were convinced that Victorian and Edwardian London remained 'out of step politically [and] not much affected by the radical movements of the century, or, for that matter by the main thrust of the Industrial Revolution'.[1] In terms of control of the environment and maintenance of public health, relatively recently created bodies in the capital frequently found themselves having to cooperate with 'pre-modern' institutions established in the seventeenth, eighteenth and early nineteenth centuries. This random mix of the old and new gave rise to a system — or, as many called it, an 'anti-system' — characterized by unparalleled governmental complexity. The Metropolitan Board of Works (MBW) and (after 1889) the London County Council (LCC), the City, the Metropolitan Asylums Board (MAB), Poor Law authorities, voluntary hospitals, the Thames and Lea Conservancy Boards, the Port of London Authority (PLA): each was individually or jointly responsible for an astonishingly convoluted body of legislative and administrative practice.

Until 1904 regulation of the eight private water concerns rested with the notoriously prejudiced company engineers, the Registrar-General's Office (RGO), the Local Government Board (LGB) and the semi-official metropolitan water analyst, the most influential of whom was the distinguished chemist, Sir Edward Frankland.[2] Parks and open spaces were individually or jointly controlled by the Crown, the MBW, the LCC, miscellaneous trusts and charities and private individuals or groups of individuals. The task of applying sanitary legislation at local level might appear to fall to the vestries, and, after 1900, the boroughs. But in many spheres – inspection of factories and workshops, prosecution of purveyors of adulterated food, anti-smoke measures and the 'protection of infant life' – responsibility was divided with the MBW in control until 1889, and afterwards the LCC. Little wonder that, confronted by so impenetrable an institutional jungle, reformers repeatedly resorted to the generalized rhetoric of democratic accountability. Castigating the practice of nomination rather than direct election, they insisted that nothing less than a restructuring of the London government system would bestow unity or coherence on day-to-day life in the capital. According to this ubiquitous discourse, the power of the vestries and their successor-bodies – the boroughs – must be radically reduced, thereby making it possible to secure standards as high as those assumed to be in place in urban provincial England.[3] Taken as a whole, metropolitan administration appeared to conform to heavily loaded images of amateurism combined with an antediluvian contempt for the spirit of representative control.

This critique was linked to the notion, invariably owing more to the cadences and logic of progressive rhetoric than demographic or epidemiological reality, that poverty and disease were persistently and at times traumatically present in the late nineteenth and early twentieth century capital. Recent research has confirmed that between the 1680s and the 1760s London constituted a desperately unhealthy environment. Repeated outbreaks of smallpox and fever struck down adults and rampant gastro-enteritic infections, convulsions, pneumonia and bronchitis triggered exceptionally high levels of infant and early childhood mortality.[4] However, from the late eighteenth century onwards, local environmental reform, increased access to rudimentary medical care and partial domestication of childhood infections led to a significant reduction in death-rates in every age-group.[5]

Following two generations of improvement, the second quarter of the nineteenth century witnessed a pronounced deterioration, a development which was almost certainly closely linked to unprecedented levels of in-migration, severe infrastructural shortcomings and increased levels of pollution. Epidemiological regression was experienced throughout urban Britain during this period though London was significantly less severely affected than newly industrializing towns in the midlands and north.[6] Nevertheless, and despite the capital's relative advantage, many mid-century metropolitan commentators were gloomily convinced that there might be a return to the desperate conditions that had prevailed between the 1680s and the 1760s. In the event cholera, typhus, typhoid, smallpox and influenza failed to gain a permanent foothold in the capital, and by the early 1870s public health activists were beginning cautiously to predict that London would never again experience the slaughter associated with this earlier era of exceptionally high epidemic mortality.

Compared with other major European cities and many other towns in Britain in the later nineteenth and early twentieth century the capital was a relatively healthy city. However − and this also greatly strengthened the progressive case − well-to-do districts frequently contained large pockets, in fact very large pockets, of abject poverty. Thus in late nineteenth century Kensington some of the very richest of Londoners lived no more than a stone's throw away from some of the most miserably deprived. In comfortable Wandsworth in the early 1870s, the unhealthy Clapham sub-district registered a population density of approximately 18 persons per acre compared to a figure of less than ten for the rest of the area.

During the same period in suburban Camberwell, St George's sub-district recorded a population density of more than 75 individuals per acre, while the figure for the suburb as a whole was no more than 25. Twenty years later, Hackney Wick − notorious throughout the late nineteenth and early twentieth centuries for squalor, substandard housing and lack of access to social infrastructure – registered a mean infant mortality rate of 263: the comparable figure for the more affluent and socially stable Hackney sub-district declined to 122.[7] During that same decade of the 1890s Shirley Forster Murphy, the first medical officer to the London County Council, initiated a series of investigations into poor and socially deprived areas in north Kensington, Holborn, Fulham, Lambeth and Rotherhithe and concluded that in localities in which 'administration [was] lax', only radical intervention would 'prevent the conditions of life falling to a point where they may endanger the safety of the whole community'.[8] In these areas, medical officers frequently sided with the LCC and the LGB in an attempt to persuade their pay-masters to give a higher priority to effective public health and environmental intervention. Temporary alliances of this kind may be detected in Southwark in 1893 and Rotherhithe, Fulham and Lambeth in 1895.[9]

In Kensington in 1898 the medical officer, Thomas Orme Dudfield, strenuously supported the LCC's attempt to compel his vestry to take 'special action' in relation to the desperately poor Notting Dale area.[10] Local opposition to reform could be intense. In 1896 Holborn found itself rebuked for employing a wholly inadequate sanitary staff, under-investing in domestic refuse services, and failing to provide alternative accommodation for individuals whose homes had been subjected to compulsory disinfection. The vestry stonewalled and it was only following additional veiled threats on the part of the LCC and the LGB that a kind of victory – in the form of the appointment of a single additional sanitary inspector – was finally achieved.[11]

Yet these deprived areas only very rarely dragged district death-rates down to the deplorable levels experienced in the most environmentally insalubrious of new industrial towns in the midlands and north. Certainly, the worst affected sectors of the capital – densely overcrowded districts in the East End and immediately to the south of the river – were devastated by cholera in 1831–2, 1848–9 and 1854–5.[12] During the second of these outbreaks, Rotherhithe was nearly as savagely afflicted as Merthyr Tydfil, widely believed to be the most polluted town in Britain. Five years later, Bermondsey experienced the highest death-rate in Britain but London as a whole escaped with mortality approximately nine times lower than that recorded in its own most heavily hit inner southern districts.[13] During the final epidemic in 1866, it was again a metropolitan district – Stepney – which recorded the highest death-toll in urban Britain. The capital as a whole now escaped with much lower mortality than Swansea, Liverpool or Exeter.[14]

Cholera made no more than a minor contribution to long-term death rates. But, despite progressive protestations to the contrary, other indicators confirmed that London's health record was significantly superior to that of the great majority of newly industrialized towns. Thus during the 1850s adults in Blackburn, Hull, Liverpool and Sheffield were between 20 and 50 per cent more likely to die from typhus than their counterparts in the capital.[15] A generation later, only Bristol, Birmingham and Bradford recorded lower typhoid death rates than London.[16] During this same period, infants in Leicester, Hull, Birmingham and Norwich were between one and three times more likely to succumb to summer diarrhoea than those born in the capital and mortality from all causes within this most vulnerable age-group was significantly lower in London than the great majority of newly industrialized centres.[17] Thus in no year between 1840 and 1910 did infant mortality in any single metropolitan district rise above that registered in the worst provincial city.[18] The most revealing index of all – life expectation at birth – certainly indicates that many towns made significant progress between 1870 and 1900. However, Londoners born in 1891–1900 could still expect to live for eight years longer than Mancunians, six years longer than Liverpudlians and two years longer than inhabitants of Birmingham. (Among a representative sample of cities with populations of more than 100,000 only Bristolians – with a life expectancy of 47, three years higher than the figure for the capital, and a year above the national average – enjoyed a superior level of health.) [19]

Nevertheless, and despite the detailed findings of broadly optimistic social, statistical and epidemiological investigations, a widely canvassed contemporary perception of London life continued to be one of unremitting poverty and disease. The unprecedented scale and uniquely complex social, economic and spatial configuration of the capital provides a partial explanation for this contradiction. In addition, a massive body of documentary and fictional literature devoted to the 'rediscovery' of poverty in the capital between 1870 and the outbreak of World War I did indeed incontrovertibly reveal scandalously sub-standard conditions in the East End and the inner southern and central districts. As has already been noted, these accounts confirmed the ubiquitous proximity of outright deprivation to 'comfort' in 'respectable' parts of the city.[20] In addition, wretchedly adverse living conditions may have been more visibly prominent in the capital than elsewhere: provincial districts characterized by extreme poverty might contain 5,000 people, but in the capital they often housed, or failed adequately to house, four times that number.[21]

These bleak communal archipelagos of economic and social backwardness in a city which claimed to be the most materially advanced that the world had ever seen generated a massive body of work devoted to anti-urbanism and the utopian fantasy of dispatching the most impoverished inhabitants of the capital to an under-populated countryside. The allure of social Darwinistic theories predicting biological collapse among 'residual' sectors of London's working-class became part of the *lingua franca* of the metropolitan intellectual elite: and as a result the capital, rather than urban provincial Britain, established itself as a primary focus for a fear of city life which both reflected and reinforced anxiety centred on the perceived economic and military decline of the nation as a whole.[22]

A kind of environmental revolution?

Recent research suggests that metropolitan historians should be less preoccupied with deeply ingrained depictions of the environmental and administrative 'backwardness' of the capital than explanations of how London developed into so relatively healthy a capital city. Such an approach brings the demographic into closer proximity with the political while simultaneously drawing attention to the extent to which the municipal idea, *sensu stricto*, may or may not have been relevant to the needs of the metropolis. It also allows us to interrogate the achievements of provincial administrations underwritten by self-consciously progressivist ideologies. In order to clear the ground for an examination of these issues, there is a need for an outline account of administrative and institutional change in London between the mid-nineteenth century and the 1920s.

Centralized and local expenditure on sewers, street cleaning and what David Owen has felicitously termed the 'miscellaneous duties' of London government depended heavily on increased supplies of water.[23] From mid-century onwards, reformers concentrated more intensively on the 'water question' than on any other issue.[24] Depicted as corrupt, profit-maximizing bodies, the companies, operating under a body of private act legislation reaching back to the seventeenth century, became massively unpopular in the aftermath of the cholera epidemics of 1848–9 and 1854–5. Thereafter, technical improvements in terms of the selection, storage and filtration of water appeared to ensure Londoners of a less polluted supply. But in 1866 extreme and culpable incompetence on the part of the East London Company triggered a cholera epidemic which killed over 4,000 inhabitants in the East End and inner north-eastern suburbs.[25] By the mid-1870s, however, the capital was receiving a greatly improved service. Goaded by a plethora of hard-hitting official and semi-official technical reports, the companies began to operate more reliable storage, filtration and delivery systems.[26] Sceptics continued to advocate the abandonment of the Thames, insisting that the capital must seek out non-river water in the Surrey hills.

In the event, during the final 30 years of the century the single most sensitive indicator – the 'typhoid index' – confirmed that London was significantly less susceptible to the infection than most other cities in Britain and Europe. In addition, differentials in the rate of mortality from the 'autumn fever' in affluent and poor districts, which had been prominent in the 1850s and 1860s, narrowed between 1870 and 1900.[27] Controversy continued to rage around the issues of constant supply and large variations in city-wide consumption. Yet reformers who deeply distrusted the companies found themselves refuted by the mortality statistics. Epidemiologists and specialists in the fields of waterworks technology and the treatment and disposal of sewage had demonstrated that it was possible to subject river water to routine purification up to a point at which it would no longer pose a severe threat to public health.[28] The companies continued to treat working-class consumers with arrogant indifference but public opinion, and surveillance on the part of a progressive scientific community, ensured that the capital was now moderately well protected against cholera, typhoid and dysentery. The MBW and the LCC repeatedly attempted to buy out the companies, but made little progress until the beginning of the twentieth century. When the private concerns were finally deprivatized and placed under the control of the Metropolitan Water Board in 1904, the recently created boroughs secured what supporters of the LCC considered to be blatant over-representation.[29] As we shall see, in relation to city-wide public utilities, deeply imbedded fears of rejuvenated Chadwickian centralization were repeatedly rekindled.

These developments were paralleled by the evolution of institutional means of reducing the incidence of disease. Nineteenth century Londoners were quite correct to be suspicious of the medical profession: doctors were able to provide relief for no more than a small number of ailments. However, the city-wide isolation system, the Metropolitan Asylums Board, established in 1868, and accessible to non-pauper patients from the 1870s, played a significant role in reducing the out-reach of epidemics of typhus, typhoid, smallpox and scarlet fever.[30] Voluntary hospitals may also have contributed to a reduction in mortality and morbidity. Formally, charters forbade the admission of individuals suffering from infectious conditions. But regulations were frequently breached. Examination of hospital registers confirms that an increasing proportion of the metropolitan population now either had access to a bed – or to out-patient treatment – for a wide range of infectious and non-infectious conditions. By the 1860s, London, with 16 per cent of its population ending his or her days away from a normal place of residence, was the most heavily medicalized city in the world. Forty years later, one third of all metropolitan inhabitants died in a voluntary or isolation hospital, Poor Law infirmary or charitable institution.[31]

At the same time, a rapid growth in applied scientific, medical, environmental and statistical knowledge injected a degree of order and rationality into the daily activities of bodies responsible for the maintenance of public health and the protection of basic environmental standards. The establishment of the General Registry Office in 1837 enhanced awareness of differentials in the incidence of disease according to locality and cause. Just as the construction of city-wide public works in the 1850s and 1860s encouraged vestries and district boards to concentrate more intensively on bolstering the quality of social infrastructure, so the growing sophistication of the GRO's annual and decennial reports exerted a highly positive influence over epidemiological surveillance within individual sanitary areas.[32]

In the mid-1850s, medical officers frequently compiled annual reports which did little more than recycle the GRO's quarterly tables of births, marriages and deaths. This continued to be the case in poorer localities until the mid-1870s. A clear majority of late nineteenth and early twentieth century districts recruited their medical officers at the lowest possible, part-time or piece-rate salaries.[33] However, in a handful of genuinely progressive areas quite different priorities prevailed. There might be strong local political opposition to the assiduously argued specialist critiques of Thomas Orme Dudfield in Kensington, John Tripe in Hackney and Shirley Forster Murphy in St Pancras. But between the 1870s and 1890s the publication of the annual report of the medical officer developed into an important event in the vestry calendar. In Kensington and Hackney annual mortality statistics were broken down into even more detailed categories than those used at the GRO. By the 1880s progressive districts were setting the pace. Intercommunicating with the GRO, exchanging information at meetings of their professional association and at the Epidemiological Society, and publishing in the *British Medical Journal* and *Lancet*, the new body of professions became integral to the London government system. Participating in the proceedings of the Chemical, Meteorological and Statistical Societies, and the Royal Society of Arts, medical officers exchanged policy-oriented bodies of knowledge and expertise.[34]

In the fields of waterworks technology, sewage treatment and disposal, as well as the identification of sources of infection associated with unsafe food and drink, local sanitary bureaucracies cooperated closely with public health specialists and epidemiologists who had served an apprenticeship with John Simon at the Medical Office of the Privy Council between 1858 and 1871, and who were now undertaking inspectorial work on behalf of the Local Government Board.[35] As with infrastructural investment, so also in terms of specialist knowledge, London enjoyed a head-start of about 20 years over a clear majority of urban provincial centres. Lest this seems too sanguine an interpretation, it is worth recalling that, in his history of metropolitan public health administration published in 1907, Henry Jephson concluded that the legislation of 1855 had:

> put a term to the chaos of local government in 'greater London' and swept away the three hundred trumpery and petty existing local bodies. It created a legally recognisable metropolis defining its component parts and boundaries. It established a definite system of local representative government in that metropolis for the administration of its local affairs. It conferred upon the new authorities not only the powers vaguely possessed and imperfectly, if at all, acted upon by their predecessors, but a considerable number of new ones. It laid the basis for the sanitary supervision of the inhabitants of greater London.[36]

Jephson also conceded that the ignominious collapse of the MBW amid well attested accusations of rigged building contracts and back-handers marked an 'unfortunate ending to a great public body which had done really great service to London'.[37] Thirty years later as sceptical an observer of the London scene as W.A.Robson readily acknowledged the scale of infrastructural progress between the 1850s and 1880s.[38] The official historians of the LCC, Gwilym Gibbon and Reginald Bell, ritually condemned the MBW as a 'glorified works contractor' but then praised its environmental legacy as 'a distinguished array of improvements that had altered the face of London and brought light and cleanness into many of the foulest haunts of disease'.[39]

Numerous other progressives lauded the performance of London's first semi-centralizing administrative authority. But the vestries were invariably treated with contempt. 'The great masses of the working classes', Jephson claimed, '... were by the deliberate decision of the great majority of [these bodies] deprived of the protection which Parliament had devised and provided for their sanitary and physical well-being'. Moreover, 'the great bulk of the local authorities deliberately ignored the remedy devised by Parliament, and with most reprehensible callousness let the evils go on and increase: ... the name "Vestry" had become almost synonymous with incapacity'.[40]

To the arch-rationalizer Sir Ughtred Kay-Shuttleworth, the inefficiency and corruption of London's local governing bodies reflected and reinforced a quasi-medieval administrative and spatial confusion. In 1878 he asked a 'typical' M.P. to imagine that he was making his way:

> from Old Palace Yard, first to the Horticultural gardens, and, then, say, to Kensal Green Cemetery. He would first pass first through the district of St John's, Westminster, St Margaret's, Westminster, St George's, Hanover Square, Chelsea and Kensington, when he would come back to St Margaret's, Westminster. In his walk ... he would pass through the vestry districts of St Margaret's, Westminster, and Paddington, enter Chelsea again, near Kilburn; and, on reaching Kensal Green, find himself in Kensington again.[41]

To Kay-Shuttleworth, all this implied nothing less than irremediable functional incompetence. It was therefore imperative that amateurish London vestries should subject themselves to reeducation and learn from what 'provincial corporations do for their own municipalities ... employ first-rate officers instead of the mere surveyors now employed; and do everything on a uniform ... system'.[42] Tried without benefit of jury, the vestries were found guilty of sabotaging rather than creatively contributing to London's nineteenth century environmental revolution. A long-drawn out appeal is still being heard: but revisionist scholarship has already established that the original trial must have been rigged.[43]

Metropolitan exceptionalism revisited

Compared with the capital, many towns and cities in England were faced by problems which ensured that an erosion of the health divide would only be slowly and unevenly achieved. New manufacturing centres paid a disproportionate price for being recent rather than anciently established large-scale urban communities. Since the beginning of the eighteenth century, and much earlier, London had suffered and adapted to numerous near-catastrophes. Crises in the relatively recent past – the Great Fire, the epidemiological set-backs of the 'hard' eighteenth century, the cholera and fever panics of the 1840s and 1850s – had seemed to many to threaten the very existence of the capital. Nevertheless, intermittent and extreme disequilibrium repeatedly gave way to a degree of stability, suggesting that the emergence of a late eighteenth century spatial and demographic critical mass may have played an important enabling role in cyclically reestablishing social and ecological balance.

London, in other words, derived hard-won gains simply from its long experience and recovery from numerous crises over a period of centuries rather than mere decades. Differential demographic growth rates in the early nineteenth century were also central to the maintenance of the metropolitan–provincial divide. Although the population of the capital expanded at just over 2.5 per cent per annum during the peak period of national urbanization between 1801 and 1841, this was a low figure when compared with increases recorded in Bradford, Liverpool, Glasgow, Manchester, Wolverhampton and Leeds, each of which experienced a growth rate of between 5 and 10 per cent. In a number of cases – Bradford, Liverpool and Glasgow – comparisons with conurbations in the contemporary developing world are far from irrelevant.[44]

Excessively rapid demographic expansion – and massive levels of in-migration – ensured that incremental, adequate consolidation of infrastructure was inherently unlikely to be secured in a city like Manchester, which grew from around 2,500 in the mid-seventeenth century to 95,000 in 1801, and no fewer than a third of a million in 1851.

The capital also derived clear-cut advantages from an exceptionally early movement towards mass suburbanization.[45] In some historical circumstances over-rapid decentralization can lead to temporary infrastructural instability: as already noted, every late nineteenth century metropolitan suburb contained within its borders over-crowded and poverty-prone sub-districts which continued to record death rates significantly above the mean for the larger areas in which they were located. Nevertheless, the decline in population densities associated with the astonishingly rapid post-1850 expansion of city-sized localities such as Lambeth, Wandsworth, Lewisham and Hammersmith greatly reduced mortality from viral and bacterial droplet infections and made a decisive contribution to improvements in life expectancy for every age-group. In addition, London's status as an imperial city played a decisive role in ensuring that it maintained a clear health advantage over urban provincial Britain. During one of the most serious environmental crises of the century – the so-called 'Great Stink' on the Thames in 1858 – members adopted a wide range of attitudes towards municipal self-government and metropolitan exceptionalism. In the event, the House voted in favour of immediate intervention. The Metropolitan Board of Works was empowered to borrow up to £3 m at 4 per cent: this would be guaranteed by the government and the principal repaid by means of a sewer rate of threepence in the pound. The decision constituted a silent revolution in relations between the national executive and the MBW, as well as a subtle sea-change in dominant provincial perceptions of the capital.[46]

In voting for the principle of metropolitan exceptionalism, members had tacitly lent their support to what Norman Davies has identified as the ideological construction of an Anglocentric 'British Imperial Isles'.[47] Furthermore, provincial representatives who questioned the wisdom of allowing London to spend money on so lavish a scale tended to deprecate increased social investment wherever it might be located. In deploring metropolitan extravagance, they also deplored levels of expenditure that might have made provincial cities safer places in which to live. Within this larger political context, the local government 'revolution' of 1835 can only have played a minor role in enabling communities to engage more effectively with large-scale environmental and public health problems. Preexisting traditions, which benefited privileged interest groups determined to maintain the political *status quo*, proved remarkably resilient. Eighteenth century improvement trusts and commissions were in any case widely believed to be doing an adequate job for a minimum of public money.[48]

Councillors vehemently opposed what appeared to them to be excessively ambitious and costly projects. Fiery radical denunciation cut across and complicated what might otherwise have constituted politically neutral debates about which tasks required immediate attention in over-crowded and deprived cities and townships. Thus in the eyes of Owenites, Chartists and independents, the deodorization and disposal of sewage emerged as explicitly ideological issues. In an environment in which there continued to be widespread support for the Benthamite orthodoxy that private contractors should undertake public works for individual localities, the spectre of businessmen growing fat on profits derived from transporting human waste to neighbouring farms, alienated radicals and economizers alike.[49] As Simon Szreter has emphasized, even when councillors agreed that a specific urban problem should be given absolute priority, deep ideological divisions invariably worked against meaningful collective action. Only in the politically more stable 1860s would the economy-obsessed middle- and lower-middle classes finally demonstrate a willingness to contemplate increased expenditure out of the rates on public works and services designed to benefit every member of the community.[50] The gradual emergence of 'united fronts' of this kind proved to be greatly more significant than the precise historical moment at which a city adopted, or failed to adopt, the 'democratic' Municipal Corporations Act.

Nevertheless, as we have already noted, provincial centres with populations of over a hundred thousand made impressive progress during the final thirty years of the nineteenth century: the four-year advantage enjoyed by the capital in terms of life expectancy at birth in 1850 had narrowed to two or three by the beginning of the twentieth century. The process whereby outer suburban metropolitan suburbs gained an advantage over all others in London was replicated outside the capital. Analysis of this issue is complicated by the fact that the registration districts comprising the largest cities in England were invariably few in number, giving the impression that each locality was divided into a unitary core and a unitary suburbanizing hinterland. But this evidential problem does not invalidate the larger picture.

Between 1871 and 1900 life expectation at birth in Sheffield improved from 35 to 39: the rise in salubrious Eccleshall was from 42 to 46. Manchester experienced an increase of four years, from 32 to 36: in leafy Chorlton-cum-Hardy the rise was from 38 to 42. Socially and economically deprived Liverpool increased from 28 to 30: 'comfortable' West Derby (Liverpool) progressed from 39 to 41.[51] During the period in which urban provincial England was narrowing its long-standing health deficit in relation to the capital, manufacturing centres in the midlands and north were themselves undergoing a similar process of internal demographic and epidemiological differentiation. However, nearly half a century might separate adoption of the Municipal Corporations Act and a partial closing of the metropolitan–provincial health divide. Little if any synchronicity is detectable between the formal democratization of urban governmental structures and measures rendering provincial centres significantly less dangerous places in which to live. In terms of health status in the period between the mid-nineteenth century cholera crisis and the outbreak of World War I, 'backward', 'irrational' and 'amateurish' London gained and maintained a slowly narrowing lead. Differentially reformed and infrastructurally modernizing urban provincial Britain struggled to close the gap.

Complicating the revisionist agenda

With a population of two and half million in 1851 and over eight million in the 1920s, London had always been far too populous to be governed by a single centralizing authority. Pondering this point – and the extent to which the capital now comprised a constellation of city-sized communities – an anonymous observer recorded in 1909 that:

> only five of the boroughs have less than one hundred thousand inhabitants: sixteen between one and two hundred thousand; five between two and three hundred thousand, and three over three hundred thousand. Thus enclosed within the metropolitan area are a number of administrative bodies equal to most of the largest provincial towns.[52]

Sixty years earlier, Edwin Chadwick had been convinced that it would be necessary to replace traditional forms of metropolitan administration with a crown-appointed commission possessing a right to overrule parish elites, deprivatize the water companies and construct a main drainage system predicated on the controversial though by no means wholly misguided principle of arterial circulation. When Chadwick was ousted from the Commission of Sewers and the General Board of Health and then symbolically drummed out of the capital, untrammeled localism failed to reestablish itself. Far from making the world safe for the vestries, the subsequent impassioned mid-century debate paved the way for compromise rather than regression or full and immediate municipalization.

Building on the environmental insights underlying Chadwick's vision of an idealized sanitary city, the MBW coordinated the construction of a massively ambitious intercepting sewage system. In doing so, the Board made it impossible for vestries and district boards to evade at least a degree of cooperation with a new and quasi-centralising authority. Denigrated both by contemporaries and successive generations of historians for its gerontocratic ineptitude and corruption, the MBW may now be more realistically assessed in the light of what it achieved between the late 1850s and the late 1880s. Here there was broad contemporary agreement that later nineteenth century London witnessed nothing less than an environmental revolution: even those who insisted that the MBW must be replaced as rapidly as possible by a directly elected and fully centralizing authority possessing comprehensive powers in the fields of public health and environmental control failed to marshal evidence to controvert such a view.

As yet too little research has yet been undertaken into the micro-politics of day-to-day administration at local level in the capital between the 1860s and 1920.[53] However, no vestry or borough conformed to the caricature of amateurish and corrupt non-interventionism rhetorically circulated by metropolitan and provincial progressives. It is now known that, following a temporary setback during the second quarter of the nineteenth century, the capital experienced an era of renewed environmental and epidemiological progress: advances were achieved in a political climate in which central control over vestries and boroughs remained semi-formal rather than legislatively compulsory. Indeed, only in the 1890s – a period of high ambition on the part of the newly established LCC – would a potentially city-wide body, armed with relevant powers, briefly succeed in monitoring and pressurizing 'backward' districts.

As we have seen, these detailed Public Health Department reports identified serious shortcomings at sub-district level in nearly every region of the capital. They also confirmed that it was unlikely that progress would be maintained unless reforming medical officers tacitly collaborated with the LCC and the LGB to convert low-spending authorities to the idea that universally positive benefits could be derived from increased expenditure on environmental infrastructure and personnel. In time, however, the Conservative government, capitalizing on its national political and ideological supremacy, undermined the LCC's universalistic project to play an ever larger role in the day-to-day administration of the largest city in the world. For their part, the vestries demanded that they be transformed into autonomous boroughs: the LGB reneged on its earlier commitment to semi-enforced metropolitan reform and encouraged the newly constituted authorities to declare what amounted to unilateral independence from the standard-setting LCC. At the same time, economic considerations proved decisive. As the Progressive T.J. Macnamara noted, the creation of the boroughs had less to do:

[with increasing] the dignity of local authorities [than] to enable the rich to slate off their obligations to the poor. The rich with their few needs want to cut themselves adrift from the poor parishes with their low rateable value and many needs.[54]

By the beginning of the twentieth century the political situation in London was no less complex than it had been in 1850. Formally, the struggle for the representative principle had been only partially successful. In 1855 the local government electorate in the capital had been approximately 195,000, or about 30 per cent of the total male population aged 20 and over. Forty years later, a million Londoners possessed the right to vote for two LCC councillors from each of the 60 metropolitan parliamentary divisions. In 1918 the Representation of the People Act increased the size of the electorate, so that by 1920 just over a million and a half inhabitants were authorized to vote in LCC elections. Comparable figures for the metropolitan vestries and boroughs rose from approximately 700,000 during the mid-1890s to about 800,000 just before the outbreak of war, and over a million and a half by 1920.

However, by this latter date, only about half of the total adult metropolitan population possessed a legislatively legitimated right to play a full role in the political life of the capital.[55] To progressives this represented near-failure and a betrayal of the mission to transform a generalized progressive impulse into the hard currency of effectively centralizing political and administrative power. Now, in the mid-Edwardian era, the massively self-confident advocate of capital-wide reform of the 1890s had degenerated into a weakened and strategically confused authority which was frequently pushed to the very margins of legislative and executive influence. The Council's 14 members on the Metropolitan Water Board were decisively outnumbered by 27 spokesman nominated by the boroughs. Representation on the Thames and Lee Conservancy Boards amounted to no more than a paltry three out of 28 and two out of 15 respectively. Ten City-influenced river interests held the whip-hand on the eighteen-member Port of London Authority, with the Council being entitled to no more than four coopted votes. The LCC would continue to be excluded until 1929 from the Metropolitan Asylums Board, which was administered by 55 members selected by the Boards of Guardians and 18 nominated by the newly created Ministry of Health.[56] Notable progress in the fields of education, transport and housing notwithstanding, the Council was rebuffed whenever it attempted to gain statutory power to intervene in boroughs which failed to meet minimum requirements under public health legislation, or to reprimand under-achieving bodies responsible for the generalized protection of the metropolitan environment.

All this carries important lessons for the metropolitan historian. Firstly, a continuing preoccupation with the minutiae of the 'London government problem' reveals so much but no more about the dynamics of daily political and social life in the capital during the late nineteenth and early twentieth century. Secondly, the achievements of the LCC – and more specifically the extent to which it fulfilled the ambitions of the founding-fathers of the late 1880s and early 1890s – have now been fully and convincingly documented.[57] These interwoven themes – the introduction of a 'rational' system of metropolitan administration and the creation of a genuine and genuinely radical city-wide authority – were themselves rooted in common political and cultural concerns: reforming the governmentally unreformable, rationalizing the irrational, and creating a materially and ethically regenerated metropolis. Thus, in terms of text and sub-text, what Mill, Jephson, Kay-Shuttleworth, W.A. Robson and other highly articulate progressives said and wrote about London had less to do with a real capital in real time than an imagined capital in unreal time. All this implies that metropolitan history should now concern itself less with formally political than explicitly cultural approaches to the evolution of economy, society, environment and collective *mentalité* in the late nineteenth and early twentieth centuries.

Third, by the outbreak of World War I, a clear majority of metropolitan boroughs were in the process of further consolidating the achievements of vestries which had themselves long since attained a high degree of institutional and bureaucratic maturity: London had finally evolved into a semi-municipalized city. At the same time, other elements of the administrative system – the Metropolitan Water Board, the Port of London Authority, the Thames and Lea Conservancy Boards – remained proudly and obstinately 'pre-modern', although no less functionally competent and in a clear majority of cases more functionally competent than their counterparts in urban provincial Britain. In terms of the dynamics of early twentieth century metropolitan government, the evidence points to a ubiquitous tension between the drive for increased professional and technical competence on the part of these non-representative bodies and continuing demands for public control championed by the LCC and some though by no means every borough.

As in the later nineteenth century, so now in the early twentieth, informal networking between the capital's scientific, medical and epidemiological elites and those who worked for committees and individuals at local level and for the independent, quango-like bodies discussed in this chapter, repeatedly saved the London government system from self-inflicted paralysis. Here, certainly, the coordinating role of the LCC – an astonishingly large, indeed profligate employer of free-floating 'experts', able to take a distanced view of the effectiveness of a thousand and one interventions at every tier of an intensely complex set of administrative structures – may well have been decisive.

Finally, recent scholarship has confirmed that the indisputable achievements of the Metropolitan Board of Works, the vestries and the boroughs constitute a retrospective refutation of the caricatured image of ineptness and corruption so expertly and persuasively constructed and rhetorically naturalized by successive generations of progressive reformers and historians. Now, more than ever, the task is to complete the revisionist agenda by undertaking detailed research into relations and structural and ideological contradictions between the 'modern' and the 'pre-modern' in the capital during the twentieth century as a whole.[58] Such work will be likely to throw light both on London's recent history and the multi-faceted and ever-shifting nature of the metropolitan–provincial divide.

PART 2

POLLUTION AND THE BURDENS OF URBAN-INDUSTRIALISM

CHAPTER 6

POLLUTION IN THE CITY

Social and legal contexts

We live in an era in which global crisis is permanently, threateningly present. Despite that fact little work has yet been completed within the mainstream of social, economic and urban history on the origins, distribution and impact of environmental pollution in the first industrial nation.[1] Nor have the nature and extent of the dilemma in towns and cities between the mid-nineteenth and mid-twentieth centuries been systematically explored or interpreted. Compared with similar research in North America and, to a lesser extent, France, British environmental history is in this sense under-developed and methodologically immature.[2] This is surprising on a number of counts. First, research programmes are frequently influenced and at times determined by pressing contemporary concerns. Secondly, cognate disciplines – and particularly sociology and anthropology – have already begun to throw light on pollution processes as social, as well as socially constructed, phenomena.[3] Thirdly, writers in these fields are providing provisional answers to a crucial and essentially historically rooted question: how was it that, in this particular place and at this particular time, this particular environmental dilemma came, finally, to be interpreted as unendurable?[4]

In what follows the literature will be surveyed in order to illuminate relationships between urban and environmental change between 1850 and 1950. An opening section outlines the social and legal processes and traditions that partially defined urban-based pollution. This is complemented by an overview of the production, treatment and disposal of human and manufacturing waste, and the contamination of river and domestic drinking water. A fourth section is devoted to the construction of a provisional narrative of the beginnings of a 'refuse revolution'. By way of conclusion, an assessment is provided of the impact of atmospheric pollution and general chronological issues. Although attention is directed throughout to the fortunes of individual towns and cities, the approach is also ecological and systemic, emphasizing the ways in which individual localities transmitted waste material to others within the urban hierarchy. An additional and important theme is that relatively small towns frequently triggered regional environmental dilemmas that were disproportionate to their demographic status.

Pollution attributable exclusively to urban-located activities is difficult to identify. But it undoubtedly afflicted all those places in which demographic growth during the late eighteenth and early nineteenth centuries was unusually rapid, in-migration heavy and the poorest members of the community subject to exceptionally high levels of overcrowding. Manufacturing pollution – both of air and water – was also invariably present, though not necessarily as a result of effluents associated with new and dynamic sectors of the economy: traditional activities – such as mining, papermaking and dyeing – also radically undermined environmental salubrity. The unplanned proximity of mills, factories and workshops to domestic dwellings ensured that conditions of life were always likely to deteriorate from levels that had intermittently threatened to become critical during the early and mid-eighteenth century.

But there was little predictability or homogeneity. Indeed, it is precisely unexpected variations within and between urban areas which require the close attention of the environmental historian. In terms of relevant quantitative indicators, analysis of the level of infant mortality, characterized by George Rosen as a highly sensitive guide to the quality of environmental and communal life, is indispensable.[5] Thus in later nineteenth − and early twentieth-century London, Sheffield and Bradford there were clear connections between higher than average infant mortality and poorer than average access to environmental and infrastructural provision.[6]

Prolonged exposure to an industrialized environment may also in itself have played a role in sustaining levels of infant death greatly above the natural average.[7] In terms of cause-specific mortality at all ages, large-scale incidence of cholera, typhoid, dysentery and diarrhoea invariably indicated radical deterioration in the quality of water supplies, while upward seasonal shifts in pneumonia, bronchitis and asthma would in time point to dangerously high levels of atmospheric impurity. In spatial terms, adverse developments in one part of an urban community invariably had dangerous repercussions for the inhabitants of others. Like bacteria and viruses, sulphurous smoke and polluted drinking water were blind to the formal administrative subdivisions of nineteenth- and twentieth-century towns and cities. Pollution generated in a large industrial area flowed outwards to exert far-reaching though non-quantifiable effects on the inhabitants of other towns, suburbia and, increasingly, as time went on, villages and hamlets. Sometimes relatively small towns − St Helens or Widnes in the early years of the alkali industry, Swansea at the beginning of the copper-smelting boom − inflicted disproportionate damage on the regions in which they were located.[8]

In a classical article, Emmanuel Ladurie has argued that the 'microbe' played a key role in the cultural 'unification' of the known world between the fourteenth and seventeenth centuries.[9] The spatial dissemination of urban-generated pollution may have worked in a similar manner, with environmental deterioration reflecting and defining the increasing interconnectedness and indivisibility of the myriad localities that comprised nineteenth and twentieth century Britain. Simultaneously, and paradoxically, however, pollution of air and water reinforced deeply embedded tensions and hostilities *between* town and country.[10] This is best illustrated by what, until the Edwardian period, continued to be the single most significant institutional definer and reflection of environmental conflict and anxiety − the demand, in terms of a common law injunction, that a given action be formally designated a nuisance and steps taken to reduce or stabilize its intensity. The reasons for the longevity of nuisance proceedings – leveled against either an individual or a collective board – may be explained in terms of the weakness of national legislation. Thus progress between the passing of the Rivers Pollution Prevention Act of 1876 and the Rivers (Prevention of Pollution) Act of 1951 should be attributed more to the activities of joint regional river boards, first established in the 1890s, than largely inactive municipalities and sanitary authorities. (A cluster of complementary acts passed between the early 1860s and the later 1880s to protect salmon against over-fishing and polluted river water proved largely ineffective.)[11]

For the bulk of the period under review, scientists failed to agree on what constituted a polluted supply of water, or how quantitative chemical standards should be enforced on socially disparate riparian interest groups. For their part, the latter clung tenaciously to customary usage, denying that contaminated water was responsible for the transmission of disease and insisting that any form of control would traumatically undermine regional economic activity, inflicting unemployment and poverty on entire urban communities. When, from the mid-1870s onwards, a legal framework for prosecution was finally created, enforcement lay predominantly in the hands of sanitary authorities, who were themselves frequently guilty of large-scale sewage pollution, as well as being under the influence of powerful cliques of manufacturers. The marginally more active policies followed from the 1890s onwards by the river boards, mainly situated in the northern industrial areas, were based on commitment to the environmental integrity of the watershed, rather than the property rights or interests of individuals or individual urban localities. Stricter control of the pollution of rivers, whether attributable to the disposal of untreated or under-treated sewage or manufacturing effluent, represented, in that sense, a reduction in the power and influence of urban elites in relation to the use of the environment. But it also gave rise to the belief that trade was being made subservient to the rod.

With only minor, local exceptions, legal action against suspected smoke polluters was even less effective. There may have been extensive propaganda against noxious vapours and this was reflected in minor victories achieved against the chemical and related industries under successive and incremental Alkali Acts from the 1860s onwards.[12] But it was long-term technological change in relation to the production of smokeless fuel immediately before and after World War II, together with a catastrophic environmental and human tragedy – the Great London Smog in 1952 – which finally precipitated the passing of the Clean Air Act in 1956.[13] Local research in the field is meagre but only a small number of centres – Derby, Birmingham, Sheffield, Liverpool, Manchester and London – framed local acts or by-laws that annually led to the prosecution of more than a handful of offenders.[14] During the 1850s largely ineffectual regulations were introduced in the capital through the unexpected intervention of Lord Palmerston.[15] At the same time by-laws in smoky Bradford proved unenforceable;[16] and 20 years later, in Leeds, it was still very nearly impossible to obtain meaningful prosecutions.[17] The reasons for failure were clear. Even more comprehensively than in relation to the pollution of rivers, *laissez-faire* arguments – that any attempt to enforce anti-smoke legislation on to the manufacturing districts would be accompanied by the closing down of factories – neutralized reformist agendas. The widely held belief that foggy towns were prosperous, and that domestic smoke was harmless when compared with a very small number of noxious manufacturing vapours, further strengthened the non-interventionist case. To this was added the problem of inspection.

The precise origin, it was argued, of a specific black and sooty emission could only be identified if an enforcing agency were to employ police, spies or inspectors. Until the early twentieth century the last of these possibilities – a fully fledged and centralized anti-smoke bureaucracy – continued to be stridently opposed by businessmen and *laissez-faire* politicians. 'Parliament', as one commentator has noted, 'passed laws giving local authorities the power to act; the local authorities, forced to confront the polluters at close quarters in the councils and courts, wavered and passed the responsibility back to the central government. In the end, little abatement was achieved.'[18] These, then, were the legal and social contexts within which, between the mid-nineteenth and earlier twentieth centuries, farmers continued to seek injunctions against manufacturers for polluting river water that ran through their fields and landowners sued manufacturers for damage inflicted on crops, gardens and what would later come to be known as 'amenity'.

In more complex variants of the same scenario, sanitary authorities took action against other sanitary authorities, for failing to cleanse or deodorize sewage which, when it flowed downstream, made life unendurable for those forced to live too close to river banks. At a bizarre extreme, as in Birmingham during the 1870s, a landowner obtained an interim order against that municipality as a result of the latter's seeming *success* in meeting the conditions of an earlier restraint.[19] Until the very end of the nineteenth century, therefore, the socially constructed and inherently pre-industrial and anti-collectivist mechanism of nuisance law continued to a significant degree substantively to define pollution and pollutant. But it also increased rather than diminished conflict between interest groups, holding different views about the uses of nature. The concept of the nuisance – finally – directs historical attention to the role played throughout the period by displacement, or the manner in which a state of affairs deemed unendurable in one centre might be transposed in a subtly different form to another locality, geographically distant from it.

Such quasi-solutions could drag an agency responsible for an original improvement into extended conflict with another public body or bodies. The environmental history of the Thames and the London region illustrates the point. Following the crisis on the river in 1858 – the year of the so-called 'Great Stink'[20] – the Metropolitan Board of Works constructed an intercepting sewage system for the capital which deposited semi-deodorized effluent at downriver outlets at Crossness and Barking. From the late 1860s on, the inhabitants of the latter community became convinced that they were being poisoned by sewage vapour. These, and similar, complaints during the next 20 years further weakened an already insecure relationship between the MBW and another body,

the Thames Conservancy Board, which held formal responsibility for
the state of the river between Staines and the sea. In this instance, as
in many others, displacement destroyed cooperation between
agencies responsible for the smooth running of local self-government
in Victorian and Edwardian Britain, redoubled tensions between
town, country and suburbia and laid bare in the starkest possible
detail the full potential volatility of the politics of pollution. It also
juxtaposed the static, locality-based characteristics of existing
methods for the prevention of environmental deterioration against
the dynamic and ever-shifting realities of pollution in an
industrializing society.

Cleansing the towns

Nothing, except perhaps political dissidence or ingratitude on the
part of the working classes, was more loathsome to the Victorian and
Edwardian social elites than sewage.[21] This detestation of matter out
of place, together with the near-collapse of traditional, semi-
voluntary and contract-based methods of disposal, went hand-in-
hand during the 1840s and earlier 1850s with widespread fear of
potential urban implosion. Within less than a generation, however,
the panic-motivated reformist programme, associated with the
Chadwickian sanitary idea, and predicated on a vision of synchronized
interaction between public water supply and sewage disposal
systems, would be subjected to intense criticism.[22] Rivers that had
scarcely been able to sustain salmon at the beginning of the century
were, by the 1860s, being compared to open sewers. Only a minority
of medical men and epidemiologists were yet fully converted to
the germ theory of disease. But the unbearable stench of ever larger
numbers of the nation's watercourses convinced contemporaries that
it was unlikely that there were no connections at all between river
pollution and devastating epidemics of cholera, typhoid and
diarrhoea. The geographical spread of the water closet, which
would have continued to play a central role in Chadwick's flawed
system for the repurification of great towns and cities, has frequently
been held responsible for the first national crisis of the rivers.

But recent research points to different and more complex sets of chronologies and explanations.

Topographical conditions, interacting with divergent accounts of the seemingly indefinitely flexible miasmatic theory of disease, legitimated the adoption of a bewildering range of environmental solutions. In addition, institutional and economic constraints dictated that nearly every urban centre between the late nineteenth and earlier twentieth centuries was characterized by subtly different relationships between water supply, sewage disposal and preferred domestic sanitary technology. Focusing on the last of these variables, Anthony Wohl has identified 'three stages. The first was the drainage of cesspools, making them smaller, water-tight and air-tight and thus self-contained. The second step was to introduce a system of dry conservancy into the homes of the poor. Only after the water was laid on, could the w.c., the third step, be adopted.'[23] Yet, as Arthur Redford has pointed out, 'in Manchester as late as 1911, less than half of the houses had water sanitation': the remainder of the population was forced to rely on a complex mix of methods and sub-methods – pail closets, ash-boxes, midden privies and wet and dry middens.[24]

Individual towns and cities, then, followed different and asymmetrical paths towards relative environmental salubrity. A crucial relationship, and one that had been insistently underscored by the Chadwickians, was between the construction of a large-scale sewage system and the installation of a city-wide supply of water. A close fit between the two encouraged the adoption of policies predicated on the introduction of water-operated sanitary appliances: lack of synchronization led to the coexistence of the kinds of wet and dry methods that have already been mentioned. As early as 1859 Glasgow gained access to an excellent water supply piped down from Loch Katrine. But opinion within the city remained divided on medical grounds about the most desirable form of sanitary technology. In addition, timidity about the financial implications of investing in major public works delayed the construction of a sewage system. The problem was only finally resolved in 1888 when the company selected to build the city's underground railway also agreed to 'undertake a... remodelling of the sewage system at their [own] expense'.[25]

In this case, incompatibility between urban networked systems continued for nearly thirty years. In neighbouring Edinburgh, by contrast, the implementation of a programme of environmental reform had to await the emergence of a consensus in relation to the filth-impregnated meadows into which the city had traditionally drained its untreated sewage. In the event, indecision reigned supreme, until the final completion of the city's sewage system in the aftermath of World War I.[26] In Belfast, the disposal question remained unsettled for nearly a quarter of a century. An initial proposal to invest in an intervening sewage system was accepted in 1887 and the project itself completed seven years later. But, in the absence of a natural drop, and of a strong ebb tide, Belfast Lough rapidly became foully polluted. Typhoid, transmitted mainly via contaminated shellfish, intermittently raged through the city, to the extent that an official report concluded in 1906 that, in terms of the dreaded 'autumn fever', 'no other city or town of the United Kingdom equals or approaches it'.[27]

Conditions, programmes and policies in Swansea were different again. Deep drainage of the town had been started as early as 1857. But construction was exceptionally slow, with the project failing to keep pace with an explosive rate of urban expansion. Between 1867 and 1889, an area of no fewer than 5,000 acres (2,025 ha.), 'much of it innocent of sanitation', became the responsibility of the medical officer and his staff. Only in the early twentieth century would Swansea's disposal system move towards completion.[28] In Leeds interactions between social, political and technological processes from the 1840s right up until the early twentieth century were so labyrinthine as to defy meaningful paraphrase.[29] In these, and numerous other urban locations between the mid-nineteenth and early twentieth centuries, methods of sewage disposal may be revealingly characterized in terms of the social construction of technology, involving systemic and sub-systemic interactions between human and non-human actors.[30] A sanitary engineer might conceive of an ideal blueprint for the disposal of human waste in a given urban environment, but only rarely would such a plan fully cohere with existing provision of a public water supply. Nor did medically authenticated legitimation of a particular form – or mix – of sanitary technologies necessarily coincide with the engineering view of the best and most hygienic method for the disposal of town waste. In that sense, the very idea of completion might remain indefinitely problematic. An intercepting sewage system could be formally and triumphantly inaugurated, yet large sections of an urban community – and particularly working-class areas – remain ill-equipped, in terms of domestic appliances, plumbing and architectural arrangements, to be able to capitalize upon it. Rapid rates of demographic growth frequently generated additional problems in relation to disposal systems and the sub-systems that they comprised. At the political level, an initial decision to reform techniques of dealing with an intolerable waste problem might coexist with and itself further stimulate the radicalization of traditional municipal values.

But full realization of real and social costs, as well as the bewildering technicalities, associated with the building of a comprehensive system might later lead to a cooling of activist ardour. Sometimes, as Christopher Hamlin has shown in relation to smaller towns, a community might be paralyzed by the prospect of 'large sanitary works'.[31] Environmental and technical dilemmas were only rarely exclusively environmentally or technically solved: and success or failure might depend, in the final analysis, on the quality of relationship between locality and centre. If, during the second half of the nineteenth century, interactions between water supply, sewage disposal and domestic sanitary technologies were numerous and unpredictable, the development of sewage treatment was no less complex. Chadwickian-cum-Benthamite commitment to the profitable agricultural reinvestment of town waste remained hypnotically attractive until the later nineteenth century. The reasons were clear. Economy-minded municipalities deplored every form of needless waste; folk memory evoked comforting images of nightstallmen removing potentially valuable excreta from town centres to verdant meadows: a minority of towns had indeed successfully invested in progressive techniques of sewage farming. But, in larger centres, exclusively agricultural modes of disposal had long lacked credibility, with contractors having to be paid rather than paying to remove ever larger and unsaleable volumes of human waste from cesspools, middens and pits.[32]

By the later nineteenth century municipalities were increasingly aware that an injunction might at any moment demand a more efficient form of treatment than could be provided by agricultural irrigation or any other known technique. (Disillusion had already developed in relation to the plethora of patent chemical deodorizers – many of them crankish and counter-productive – that had come on to the market during the 1860s.[33]) In the 1890s expert attention turned towards biological – or bacterial – filter-bed treatment; and, within another generation, what seemed to be an even more effective aerobic process, making use of activated sludge, had been adopted in a number of towns.[34] In the longer term, however, neither the improved filter-bed, nor the activated sludge procedure, achieved technical hegemony in the quest for a means of repurifying sewage, which would approximate to an 'artificial intensification and acceleration of the ordinary aerobic processes of natural purification that go on in rivers polluted by limited amounts of organic wastes'.[35]

Landlocked Birmingham, whose drainage and pollution problems have already been touched upon, deployed the full available range of sewage treatment techniques between the mid-nineteenth and mid-twentieth centuries. Following the initial installation of sedimentation plant in the 1850s, by the 1870s the city was experimenting with lime precipitation. But volumes of sewage continued to rise and the council was next advised by experts to invest in 2,500 acres (1,013 ha) for the purpose of agricultural irrigation. Initially, unwilling to become involved in so large an outlay, the council had nevertheless, under repeated threat of legal action, purchased 1,500 acres (608 ha.) by the later nineteenth century. Thereafter land irrigation rapidly began to be replaced by bacterial beds.

During the interwar years, Birmingham, like other large centres, embraced the activated sludge procedure, only to shift back, during the 1950s, towards a mixed regime, dependent on activated sludge and alternating double filtration beds.[36] The problem might now seem to have been technologically solved: but the city was still confronted by a serious displacement dilemma in relation to the disposal of sludge. According to traditional agricultural criteria, the rule of thumb had been that 10 acres (4 ha.) were required to cleanse the sewage of an urban population of a thousand. The comparable figure for single filtration was 1 acre (0.4 ha.); for alternating double filtration, two-thirds of an acre (0.3 ha.); and for activated sludge, half an acre (0.2 ha.).[37]

During the early nineteenth century, it had been assumed that town waste could be fed directly on to the land as a means of simultaneously cleansing urban areas and boosting agricultural production. The processes – economic, technological and cultural – whereby the concept of town waste had become separated from that of an idealized agriculture had been long and confused. The uneven development of technologies for sewage treatment – culminating in the bacterial and aerobic revolution between 1890 and 1920 – redefined the ways in which sanitary engineers and public health activists conceived of relationships between technology and nature. Displacement continued throughout to be a dominant problem associated with environmental quality in urban and immediately extra-urban locations, but, precisely because they sought to mimic nature, the new aerobic techniques both redefined displacement and naturalized technological systems.

Rivers and water supplies

It is no easy task to integrate this account of sewage disposal and treatment with a narrative of changing levels of river pollution between the mid-nineteenth and mid-twentieth centuries. But the emerging consensus is that, in terms of pollution attributable to human waste, increasingly efficient disposal techniques led to a slow though regionally uneven recovery. Focusing on a single, though in many respects untypical, river – the Thames – one commentator has identified a period of deterioration between 1800 and 1850; slow and chequered improvement between 1850 and 1900; renewed decline between 1900 and 1950; and decisive renewal in the years after 1950.[38] It should, however, be borne in mind that there were no major surveys of Britain's waterways between 1915 – the year of the final report of an epic Royal Commission on Sewage Disposal, set up in 1902 – and the end of World War II.

But an investigation undertaken by the Trent Fishery Board in 1936 stated that, out of 550 miles (885 km) of river, nearly 'a quarter were lethal to all animal and plant life'.[39] This may have been predominantly attributable to the ever-increasing volume, as well as growing chemical complexity, of manufacturing effluent – in 1973 local authorities were finally required to allow such waste directly into their sewers.[40] In the early 1950s a more optimistic report stated that grossly polluted stretches of non-tidal rivers had been reduced.[41] By that date, also, fish and other forms of sensitive aquatic life not been seen in the Thames since the pre-crisis days of the 1820s finally began to return to their ancient haunts.[42] Yet, even following the passing of the Rivers (Prevention of Pollution) Act of 1951, it proved difficult to move swiftly against local authorities, still reliant on antiquated methods of sewage disposal, or manufacturers ignorant or dismissive of best existing environmental practice.

Any progressivist temptation to associate the post-war quasi-nationalization of water with more coherent and comprehensive anti-pollution measures must therefore be resisted.[43] Towards the end of the 1950s the scourge of poliomyelitis directed the glare of publicity on to seaside resorts which, since the 1870s, had sought to deal with massively increased volumes of sewage during the summer season, by building ever longer and larger outlet pipes. Astonishingly, along a coastal strip 150 miles (241 km) in length between Liverpool and Barrow-in-Furness, a 'minimum of 200,000 gallons of crude sewage was discharged per mile daily'.[44] The historical moment, therefore, at which it had finally become technologically and epidemiologically imperative to repair or replace Victorian seaside sewage systems coincided with the first environmental 'crisis of the beaches'. The state of the rivers would continue to attract official and lay attention, but by the 1960s the ever-sensitive weathervane of environmental anxiety had swung towards the displacement of raw sewage and sludge into seas and oceans.

The polio scare of the late 1950s was all the more shocking since water as a free or unusually cheap semi-public good had long been disassociated from death and disease. At the beginning of the period, there had been heavy reliance on informal sources – springs, wells and streams; indeed, some individuals claimed to prefer the taste of such supplies to those provided by the private and municipal concerns.[45] By the mid-nineteenth century, however, and more intensively during the final thirty years of the century, there was large-scale investment in public water supply systems.[46] But in terms of availability, reliability and salubrity there continued to be large differentials. (The two variables – quality and quantity – were closely linked: the smaller the amount of available domestic water, the more likely that it would be used in ways that increased rather than reduced the spread of infection.)

Thus in Edinburgh in 1872 fewer than half the houses below a value of £5 a year had access to water.[47] In Dundee, during the 1860s, supplies continued to be derived from wells 'or from barrels on carts sold at 1/2d or 1d a bucket'.[48] And in Merthyr – the most polluted town in Britain? – there was an all-out water war. For more than ten years, from mid-century on, the iron masters, coordinated by the Guests and the Crawshays, had claimed the foully contaminated Taff as their own for manufacturing purposes, while simultaneously seeking to convince the rest of the community that, as controllers of the local Board of Health, big employers should be empowered to establish a private water company. The plan was eventually stymied by parliamentary agents who reminded the iron masters that no government had yet 'granted rating powers to be used for guaranteeing profit to a commercial company'. Meanwhile, very large numbers of working-class inhabitants in Merthyr were forced to obtain their water from pools, ponds and ditches.[49]

London, which depended until 1903 on private companies rather than a single, metropolitan concern, demonstrated wide disparities. Thus, as late as the 1890s, 31 per cent of all inhabitants in the capital lacked access to a permanent supply, a figure that rose to approximately one half in working-class districts to the north and east.[50] In terms of safety, it was only during the final thirty years of the century that in the capital and elsewhere a majority of companies began to deliver a moderately reliable supply; crucial technical improvements included the construction of adequate reservoir storage capacity, more carefully selected sources of raw water and closely controlled rates of slow sand filtration. During the transitional period between 1850 and 1870, when a public supply finally replaced informal sources, it was widely and correctly believed that companies had intermittently pumped sewage-tainted water directly into the homes of their consumers.

Patterns of cholera mortality retrospectively confirmed such a view, as well as the contention that it was improvements in waterworks technology, combined with increased hygienic awareness, that had played a major role in saving Britain from the epidemiological disaster that struck Hamburg in 1892. During the final thirty years of the century, typhoid, rather than cholera, emerged as a key indicator of the extent to which a given supply might be unsafe or a water company guilty of technical ineptitude.[51] As typhoid declined, so public confidence in water as a routinely reliable commodity increased. But still there were avoidable tragedies. Even after the introduction of chlorination during World War I, there continued to be small-scale, water transmitted outbreaks of the infection; and, as late as 1937, Croydon, a pioneer of progressive sewage farming, was stricken by an epidemic traced back to faecally contaminated supplies.[52]

Smaller, non-industrial towns in the south may have delayed.[53] But, by the end of the period, the great majority of urban areas enjoyed a cheap, plentiful and salubrious supply of water. Poliomyelitis may have briefly and frighteningly reactivated fears of large-scale water-transmitted infection but it relatively rapidly yielded to medical and epidemiological delimitation. The purification of polluted supplies of drinking water had finally ensured that both the external environment and the internal micro-environment had been rendered massively more congenial, in particular, to the well-being of the most vulnerable age-groups – infants, children and the elderly.

A refuse revolution?

Changes in services for household waste also raised standards and expectations. At the beginning of the period, domestic and other refuse was either piled at a distance from dwellings or deposited in dustholes before being removed, more or less efficiently, by contractors. (The evidence frequently fails to discriminate between domestic refuse, street sweepings and sewage.) In Stirling in the late eighteenth and early nineteenth centuries, collection had been in the hands of contractors. But carting waste away from the town centre proved to be an expensive item in relation to the operation as a whole. Consequently, those who had tendered cheaply and persuasively soon began to indulge in false economies. In the early 1840s, therefore, the council decided to sack the contractors and employ direct labour. But it offered exceptionally low wages and the job continued to be badly and sloppily done. In desperation contractors were recalled.[54]

The years between the late 1840s and the 1880s are a dark age in the social history of cleansing and scavenging but the consolidating Public Health Act of 1875 allowed local authorities to cart away domestic refuse and, following further legislation in 1907, to do the same for trade waste.

Between 1880 and 1914 urban Britain may have gone through a refuse revolution. (There continued, however, to be strong though inexplicable resistance to the fixed, French dustbin.[55]) Services were believed to be more efficient in Scotland and the north than in London, where several boroughs during the interwar period continued to rely on slapdash and unhygienic contractors.[56] In this field, at least, municipal socialism was far from triumphant. As patterns of production, energy use and consumption shifted and diversified, so, also, did the structure of household waste and the contents of the typical urban dustbin. Dust itself had accounted for no less than 80 per cent of the total in one London borough in the 1890s[57] and, in 1895, an authority on the subject insisted that 'nothing is to go into the dustbin except dust, ashes and paper'.[58] By 1950, dust had been almost wholly replaced by paper, board, putrescibles and plastics.[59]

Destructors and incinerators were adopted in many towns from the Edwardian period onwards, not least in the hope that large enough quantities of heat would be generated to produce cheap supplies of public service electricity.[60] In the longer term, however, burgeoning volumes – and categories – of household refuse necessitated widespread use of landfill techniques. By the 1960s, over 90 per cent of the waste collected by all local authorities – urban and rural – was being dealt with in this way. Soon, however, yet further displacement problems, related to a chronic shortage of extra-urban land space, persuaded policy-makers to reconsider the advantages of selective incineration.[61] (Twenty years later excessive emission of dioxins would again cast doubt on the desirability of the procedure.)

Conceptualizing the smoke problem

The campaign to combat the gross deterioration of river and drinking water, coordinated by the Rivers Pollution Commissioners under the leadership of the distinguished chemist, Edward Frankland, had been mobilized in the 1860s and 1870s. Urban-based anti-smoke movements are less amenable to precise chronological definition. Concern over stench, dust and soot had first revealed itself in medieval London. In the late seventeenth century, John Evelyn presented the monarch with what would now be termed an environmental manifesto to combat atmospheric pollution. Besides transmitting a subtle ideological subtext, Evelyn's much reprinted and cited pamphlet, *Fumifugium*, established itself as a canonical document in relation to every subsequent attempt to reduce atmospheric pollution in London and elsewhere.[62] Eighteenth-century attitudes towards, as well as preventative action against, smoke remain obscure but London probably experienced a heavily soot-laden fog about once every four years during the period as a whole;[63] and poets, satirists and playwrights declaimed insistently against the atmospheric filth of the ever-expanding city – its foul trades, odours and vaporous fogs. Such discourses would stabilize an enduring cultural pattern. Domestic smoke and soot were acceptable and might even be physiologically beneficial. Specified manufacturing vapours and steam engine soot, by contrast, would need to be curbed.

In the early nineteenth century, metropolitan reformers confronted this steam engine problem and the extent to which new methods of production, as well as old and filthy trades, now endangered architecture, plant life and health. Compared with cities like Manchester, Salford and Glasgow, however, the capital still suffered only minor damage from the atmospheric by-products of manufacturing processes. In the industrial districts flakey soot floated down in huge quantities on to gardens, allotments and newly washed clothes, encouraging the establishment in Manchester of the first authentic anti-smoke pressure group. London's famous fogs, meanwhile, were visibly and permanently transforming themselves into an ominous dirty yellow. Yet official eyes were still directed obsessively downwards, intent on finding solutions to the twin and environmentally related threats of cholera and unprecedentedly contaminated streets, courts and alleys.

The Chadwickian sanitarians – not least Neil Arnott, inventor of a stove that was claimed to reduce expenditure on domestic fuel and warm rooms more efficiently – were not, however, indifferent to the problem. Developing a line of argument which would, in one or another form, be sustained until the end of the century, they insisted that solar light was an essential precondition for healthy urban existence. If it were absent, or restricted, disease and, more specifically, fever would flourish. Such an epidemiological calamity would lead to reduction in earnings and added expense for medical assistance – cumulative costs that would be further increased by 'money that the benevolent [must] subscribe to fever hospitals and other institutions'.[64] By the 1850s Chadwick himself was developing a more sophisticated variant of this kind of cost-benefit analysis and claimed that the capital's perennial winter and spring fogs involved £5 m a year in extra washing bills, or between a twelfth or thirteenth of a typical middle-class income.[65] When such debilitating meteorological episodes dramatically increased in frequency and intensity – peaking in London between the 1870s and the 1890s – similar exercises in the evaluation of environmental damage would be undertaken and given wide publicity.

The displacement effects of late nineteenth-century smoke fog, mainly attributable to the consumption of ever-increasing quantities of domestic coal, were probably less severe than those associated with a sewage-polluted river, transmitting cholera or typhoid bacteria from one urban centre to another geographically distant from it. But no such optimism was justified in relation to the appallingly damaging fall-out, and venomous riverside waste-heaps, associated with the alkali industry, centred on St Helens, Widnes, Tyneside and Glasgow.[66] In 1862, frustrated by a string of failed legal suits and restraints against the manufacturing interest, the largest landowner in the region, Lord Derby, coordinated a packed select committee. With remarkable rapidity, he gained the support of both houses for a system of inspection that encouraged less environmentally harmful, as well as more economic, methods of production.

Angus Smith, the first chief inspector (who would also later oversee the implementation of the half-hearted Rivers Pollution Prevention Act of 1876), and his successor, Alfred Fletcher, opted for a collaborative rather than confrontational relationship with the manufacturing interest. In a classic account of the Alkali Inspectorate, Roy MacLeod has discerned a six-phase progression from 'experimentation in methods and administration' during the 1860s to mature consolidation in the 1890s and the first decade of the twentieth century.[67] At the same time, however, the new bureaucracy, centred on London, Liverpool, Newcastle, Manchester and Glasgow, became aware of several structural and operational limitations. As soon as one vapour had been evaluated and partially controlled, another, the product of the ever-growing complexity of the late-nineteenth century economy, became equally threatening.

Debilitating, also, was the veto which successive Alkali Acts placed on investigation of and action against the environmentally harmful consumption of domestic fuel. Smith and Fletcher were anxious to transpose an increasingly coherent and practical body of chemical and meteorological knowledge on to the domestic smoke problem. By the late nineteenth and early twentieth centuries medical men were devoting increasing attention to the connections between adverse atmospheric conditions and the incidence of pneumonia, bronchitis and asthma;[68] and the damage done to children by an inadequate supply of sunlight and the associated scourge of rickets.[69] At an extreme, social theorists and reformers constructed deeply pessimistic linkages between perpetual fog, degenerationist and social Darwinistic anxiety, and a generalized crisis of the city.[70]

Such agendas appeared to confirm entropic obsessions, associated, on the one hand, with debates surrounding the Second Law of Thermodynamics and, on the other, with the conclusions of W. S. Jevon's disturbing *The Coal Question*, first published in 1866.[71] Environmental concern now combined with and reinforced communal disquiet over resource depletion and the sustainability of urban and, indeed, every other form of advanced civilization. Precipitated by an unprecedentedly lavish use of domestic coal, the smoke fog crisis had triggered a national debate on the possibility of absolute energy depletion. A major priority was to find ways of luring the ordinary domestic consumer away from the blazing, open hearth, and to persuade him to invest in stoves and modified grates which burnt smokeless rather than traditional, smoky coal. But the major reformist body in the field in the 1880s – the National Smoke Abatement Institution – brought to its task many of the economic and social assumptions of the aristocratic and upper middle-class elite.

It underestimated costs of conversion in relation to net disposable income, the extent to which permanent access to the 'cheerful hearth' confirmed upward social mobility and familial solidarity and the amount of extra housework that would need to be expended on laying and stoking a modern grate. A similar, though less socially exclusive, pressure group, the Manchester and Salford Noxious Vapours Abatement Association, campaigned against the continuing though typologically distinctive forms of smoke pollution which continued to bedevil the northern industrial regions.[72] An anti-smoke organization also established itself in Leeds. 'In our own inspections for three weeks', an activist there reported in 1906, 'out of 79 boiler chimneys 51 emitted black, opaque smoke for over ten minutes in the hour. Yet the convictions for smoke nuisance were ludicrously few: in one year, there was only one, and the average is three per annum, with a fine of 10s. each.'[73]

By the earlier twentieth century, then, remarkably little had been done to reduce the regular and debilitating incidence of smoke fog in either London or the great manufacturing centres. Fortuitously, however, the Edwardian era witnessed what is perhaps most accurately described as an autonomous meteorological improvement.[74] But relief was short-lived. As World War I drew to a close, the capital was again shrouded in impenetrable fog during February, 1918. Nor was there any radical improvement during the interwar years. Foggy episodes were shorter than they had been between 1870 and 1900, and fog-related deaths from bronchitis, pneumonia and asthma seemingly less numerous. But on four occasions during the 1920s, and four more in the 1930s, London was paralyzed.[75] Whether a similar pattern was reproduced in the urban north of England, and in industrial Scotland and Wales, is unclear. Prolonged depression certainly seems likely, in itself, to have produced precisely those relatively smoke-free skies that had earlier been feared and decried as symbols of communal unemployment and poverty. But, for those in work, coal was plentiful and cheap and the attractions of a roaring, and smoky, hearth no less seductive.

Observers travelling through and reporting on the state of industrial Britain during the 1930s still frequently referred to ubiquitous smoke and fog; and so, also, did pressure groups campaigning for tighter legislative control.[76] Progressives might sing the praises of clean electricity, but working-class sectors of British cities were still heavily dependent on coal for the purpose of domestic heating. In the immediate aftermath of World War II, the capital experienced yet another severe fog cycle with excess deaths reportedly rising by 800 between 27 November and the beginning of December 1948, and, astonishingly, by no fewer than 4,000 during the terrible darkness that descended on the city between 5 December and 8 December 1952.[77] These post-war smogs almost certainly contained life-damaging elements not present during comparable episodes in mid- and late Victorian Britain: medical scientists and epidemiologists in the 1950s were in possession of knowledge that had not been available to those who had sought to investigate and understand the great smoke fogs of the earlier period. In that sense, the death-toll attributable to urban atmospheric pollution over the previous 100 years had almost certainly been higher than was implied by contemporary statistical estimates. Finally, in 1956 the Clean Air Act entered the statute book. Before the legislation became fully operational 19 local authorities had established smokeless zones, and 40 more had obtained local acts to control smoke from industrial chimneys.[78] Belatedly, 150 years of anti-smoke propaganda had begun to do its work.

Environmental chronologies

Goaded by the lash of moralized sanitary ideology, the sewering and cleansing of towns and cities that had started during the 1840s would in time stabilize and then dramatically transform the urban environment during the late nineteenth and early twentieth centuries. Yet the measures directed towards that goal – the disposal and treatment of sewage, provision of a genuinely public supply of water, street cleaning and systematic removal of household refuse – gave rise to unprecedentedly grave displacement problems in a society whose systems of local self-government were incapable of reacting rapidly to socially and epidemiologically debilitating pollution of air and water. Reformist activity between the 1860s and 1890s was, therefore, simultaneously devoted to the construction of social infrastructure, and the amelioration of some at least of the evils inflicted on rivers by the cleansing of the cities in the 1840s and 1850s.

In terms of sewage disposal, large-scale systems were easier to design than build or – problematic term – complete. Continuingly rapid demographic expansion, administrative restructuring, lack of technological know-how, the vicissitudes of municipal politics – each or all of these ensured that comprehensive systems could take anything up to a generation and a half to achieve. A network of public water supply systems, without which the draining of urban areas would not have been possible, was, on the other hand, more rapidly and – in social and political terms – less problematically installed. (The repeated reactivation of the London water question between 1870 and 1900, involving acrimonious debate between rival supporters of private and metropolitan control, may have been the exception that proved the rule.)

Laggards there may have been but, between 1870 and 1914, the great majority of towns and cities gained access to water supplies that could be described, in quantitative terms, as 'adequate'. But safety, reliability and equality of access were less easily obtained and it was only after the interwar period that urban communities finally came to be exempt from occasional, and sometimes serious, outbreaks of water-transmitted infection. New forms of waterworks technologies and procedures for the treatment, rather than the deodorization, of sewage were crucial to this transformation. The bootstrap empiricism that had informed techniques of water purification during the early and mid-nineteenth century, had, by the 1890s, been refined and systematized, in the light of what was now known about biological processes underlying slow sand filtration.

As for sewage treatment, aerobic methods gradually replaced traditional procedures associated with agriculture and agricultural irrigation. As commitment to the commonsensical necessity of returning waste to the fields weakened, so new techniques – as well as, to a certain extent, the nature in which they were situated – were imaginatively and scientifically reconceptualized: fertilization was replaced by systems that imitated what really occurs when streams and rivers became moderately, though not foully, polluted. Precisely what to do with residual sludge remained – and still remains – a troubling dilemma.

These changes proceeded in a social and political framework in which national legislation, repeatedly undermined by powerful manufacturing interests, remained weak and imprecise. (Water-transmitted industrial effluent proved exceptionally difficult to identify and prosecute.) From the 1890s onwards regional river boards extended their administrative control. But compared with the Alkali Inspectorate, they lacked the power to take action against clearly specified and legislatively outlawed pollutants. Despite major successes, the Alkali Inspectorate itself continued, as we have seen, to be debarred from intervening in cases traceable to the unacceptably smoky consumption of domestic fuel. This cultural sanctity of the hearth was reinforced by the fact that epidemiological data on the incidence of pneumonia, bronchitis and asthma remained ambiguous when compared with similar bodies of knowledge, widely available from the 1870s onwards, on water-transmitted cholera and typhoid.

There are also grounds for believing that atmospheric pollution attributable to domestic smoke could only be vigorously prosecuted once both the water and noxious vapour problems had been identified and partially resolved. Successful environmental intervention may, in that sense, have depended – to borrow Mary Douglas and Aaron Wildavsky's phrase – on the 'selection' of a single, and no more than a single, environmental threat at a given historical juncture. Even when scientific and administrative scrutiny was brought intensively to bear on the domestic fuel problem, the diagnosis of coal smoke as an unquestionably noxious residue was only haltingly and unwillingly accepted. There was a significant shift in municipal opinion during the Edwardian period – years that were characterized, paradoxically, by an improvement in urban atmospheric conditions – and even more decisive change between 1918 and 1939. But it was only following the traumatic events in the capital in 1952 that the state initiated far-reaching legislative action.

Britain's still smoky towns and cities during the early 1950s may be categorized as intermediate between the blatantly polluted urban environments of the mid-Victorian period, and the invisibly threatened conurbations of our own times. When, in the early 1960s, the Clean Air Act became fully operational, many places were visually and aesthetically transformed. Yet within less than a generation, collective environmental *angst* would be reactivated. Trepidation, this time, was grounded less in the collective conviction that foul air and water would once again drag urban Britain down into squalor and decimating infectious disease, than that new and, to laypeople, bewilderingly complex chemical pollutants – the products of ever more energy-intensive patterns of production, transportation and consumption – would threaten the sustainability of late twentieth-century urban, and, indeed, global life. Similarities – as well as subtle differences – with earlier waves of environmental concern, themselves rooted in and magnified by fear of entropy and the potential collapse of advanced civilization, would soon become too striking to be ignored.

In conclusion, this overview may be seen as partially substantiating Jeffery Williamson's important argument that Britain significantly under-invested in 'city social overhead' during the earlier years of industrialization. However, as has been emphasized throughout, technical incompetence and the vagaries of local politics invariably played as important a role in inhibiting effective environmental intervention as the immaturity and rigidity of national capital markets.[79] In that sense, however brilliantly elaborated it may be, cliometric counterfactualism is no substitute for fully contextualized accounts of the environmental histories of individual towns and cities.

CHAPTER 7

'THE HEART AND HOME OF HORROR': THE GREAT LONDON FOGS OF THE LATE NINETEENTH CENTURY

Conceptualizing pollution and disease

The last 25 years have witnessed profound changes in the histories of medicine and public health. In a British context, the late Roy Porter pioneered the reconstruction of patient experiences, deliberately downplaying a venerable academic obsession with the lives and careers of great surgeons and physicians.[1] Over the same period Anthony Wohl, Anne Hardy, Nancy Tomes and Michael Worboys have interrogated Whiggish interpretations which had assumed a non-problematic transition from 'primitive' miasmatism to universal acceptance of a modern and scientific bacteriological world-view.[2] Integrating the histories of science, culture and ideology, Christopher Hamlin has demonstrated that prominent public health reformers – Chadwick, Frankland, Farr, Simon – referred to the sanitary sphere in a style which drew on discourses as heavily influenced by religious and moral as by environmental values.[3]

Finally, historical demography and epidemiology, simultaneously located within and reacting against a dominant McKeownite paradigm, have undergone conceptual and methodological transformation.[4] However, progress in the neighbouring sub-discipline of environmental history has been less impressive. In the United States Joel Tarr, William Cronon, Martin Melosi and others have championed a city-oriented variant of a sub-discipline long dominated by a deep preoccupation with wilderness.[5] In Britain, by contrast, powerfully established traditions in economic and social history have militated against the academic autonomy of a subject, which, languishing as a minority interest, remains wedded to predominantly scientific rather than unequivocally historical objectives. Outline surveys of environmental change in Britain between the eighteenth and twentieth centuries have now finally begun to appear.[6] But at the time of writing there is only one city-specific case-study of atmospheric pollution during the peak period of industrialization and hardly anything at all on communal response to the Victorian and Edwardian water problem.[7] As a consequence, very little is yet known about why at a specific historical juncture a situation long deemed acceptable came finally to be categorized as an unendurable pollution problem. Nor have researchers yet probed the ways in which non-environmental factors – for example, preexisting tensions between parties and/or influential interest groups – fed back into and galavanized environmental debate and action. Only a handful of writers have yet examined responses to pollution problems in order to reveal the nature and differences between different municipal and metropolitan regimes.[8]

This chapter links environmental history to the socio-medical approaches outlined in this introduction. The central focus is on the great smoke fogs which periodically paralyzed the capital between the 1870s and the outbreak of World War I. We begin with a brief sketch of the nineteenth century metropolitan meteorological regime. This is followed by an examination of growing mid-nineteenth century preoccupation with the calculation of the social costs of atmospheric pollution – a quintessentially Chadwickian approach to the problem of environmental degradation, influentially developed in late Victorian London by the meteorologist-cum-social reformer, F.A.R. (Rollo) Russell. This brief venture into the origins of environmental economics prepares the way for an account of changes in medical attitudes towards the impact of fog on respiratory disease and the highly moralized degenerationist framework within which the health of the people and life-threatening atmospheric pollution came to be located.

The intensity of this discourse is highlighted through textual interpretation of William Delisle Hay's popular science fiction shocker *Doom of the Great City*, which was published at the height of the metropolitan fog crisis in 1882. Perceived as a totality, these bodies of thought – economic, epidemiological and social Darwinistic – can be seen to have legitimated a catastrophist view of relationships between endemic fog and the crisis of the inner city. At an extreme, those who articulated this anti-urban ideology proposed nothing less than a real or imagined pastoralization of the greatest capital in the world.

Late nineteenth century Londoners – and particularly metro-politan professional and scientific elites – believed themselves to be endangered by an unprecedentedly severe atmospheric threat, even more potentially dangerous than the water problem that had triggered catastrophic mid-century cholera.[9] But whereas technical procedures which would eventually deliver safer supplies of public water had been understood since the 1850s, and were refined over the ensuing generation, measures to reduce the severity of the domestic smoke problem continued to be considered technically – and politically – inoperative.[10] For this and other reasons, it is contended here, terrifying images of 'strangulating' smoke fog and biological or racial decline interracted with and reinforced one another, generating an astonishingly powerful set of deeply pessimistic environmental discourses. As a consequence, incipient activism gave way to perversely self-fulfilling – and as Hay's fantasy narrative indicates – luridly sentimental *fin de siecle* despair. In the longer term partial substitution of gas for coal coalesced with autonomous meteor-ological factors to reduce the severity of the fog problem in Edwardian London. However, during the interwar era, and even more traumatically as a result of the notorious smog episode of 1952, the age-old spectre, which had first afflicted the capital in the medieval period, returned to haunt and kill vulnerable members of the metropolitan community.

Towards the dark?

Mid-eighteenth century meteorologists were convinced that the great fog of 1755, which coincided with the devastating Lisbon earthquake of that year, ushered in a new and less stable climatic cycle, characterized by increasing numbers of dense smoke fogs.[11] In the early winter of 1796 William Bent, a Strand-based chronicler of the London weather, recorded that his part of his city had been shrouded in a 'thick and dark fog [for] most of the morning'.[12] In the winter and spring of 1813–14, the distinguished medical man, Thomas Bateman noted that 'all objects at a few feet distant from the eye [were] invisible: houses, railings, streets and trees, and even the cobwebs hanging over them, became thickly spangled with ... freezing humidity'.[13] As pea-soupers increased in early nineteenth century London, accident rates soared. Coaches overturned: a girl 'missed the rising path leading to the Surrey Canal ... and fell in and was drowned': a watchman 'in the parish of Marylebone fell down [in the fog] while crying the hour and was found the next morning with his neck broken'.[14]

The pioneering Tottenham-based meteorologist, Luke Howard, confirmed that the capital experienced several severe episodes during the late 1820s.[15] In 1827 he recorded that 'between nine o'clock and midnight all movement in the city became exceptionally dangerous: flambeaux and link-boys were equally in requisition: the most brilliant gas-light could scarcely penetrate the gloom'.[16] The incidence of fog increased during the 1830s, but blanket episodes became less frequent.[17] In the 1840s, however, conditions again deteriorated and in February 1843 the weather was so bad that 'it was almost impossible to see from one side of the street to the other'.[18] Eighteen months later street and river traffic were massively disrupted and within a decade smoke fog would be 'prevalent' on no fewer than 20 occasions during the course of a single winter or spring month.[19] In 1859 *The Builder* complained that the inhabitants of the capital were now forced to endure the 'fog season' in conditions akin to semi-darkness.[20]

By the late 1850s, also, journalistic benchmarking had confirmed that midday close-downs had become more frequent, costly and dangerous. In the early 1860s dirty-white was beginning to be replaced by sulphurous yellow, with extended periods of foggy weather seriously disrupting the casual labour market in the eastern and inner city core districts.[21] Despite due warning, meteorologists, epidemiologists and urban reformers were genuinely shocked by the severity of the great crises of December 1873, January 1882, winter and spring 1886–7, December 1891, December 1892 and November 1901.[22] If conditions were bad between 1871 and 1875, they were even worse between 1886 and 1890, with nearly twice as many severe episodes recorded in the later 1880s than the early 1870s.[23] During winter and early spring in this period the capital found itself intermittently under siege – there were 55 serious occurrences a year between 1871 and 1881 and 69 between 1882 and 1892, with peaks of 86 and 83 in 1886 and 1887.[24]

In the great fog of December 1873, pedestrians in the central districts were unable to see from one side of the street to the other: 'fat cattle slumped to the ground and expired' at the Islington Great Show: breathing was 'painful and constricted': and progressive medical men became convinced that metropolitan mortality had exceeded the normal weekly average by more than 700.[25] Between November 1879 and February 1880 deaths attributed to asthma 'mounted to an unprecedented degree' and on several days 'lamp-post [s] four and a half yards distant [were] invisible at 10 a.m'.[26] The 'severe and protracted fog [which] visited London at Christmas, 1891 . . . lasted without intermission from Monday evening until Friday night, or close upon a hundred hours'.[27] 'No one', an observer wrote, 'who has once experienced a bad fog in town is likely to forget the dense, heavy, oppressive feeling of the air, and the unnatural darkness at midday that can almost be felt.'[28] Looking back from the vantage-point of 1953, the year after London experienced its most traumatic twentieth century smog episode, the veteran meteorologist L.C.W. Bonacina reminisced about similar events in the capital during the late nineteenth century. 'A really bad fog', he wrote:

> appeared early in the morning as a thick white mist, like country fog, only dirtier. With the lighting of the fires it would soon become yellow and pungent, irritating the throat and eyes, till by midday the continued outpouring of chimney products would have turned the fog a sooty brownish black causing the darkness of night. During the afternoon there might be a partial improvement to the lighter yellow phase, but following the early sunset with renewed condensation through radiation the density of the fog would be such as to bring the street traffic to a standstill.[29]

Revisiting the sense of chaos generated by metropolitan 'darkness at noon', Bonacina went on to evoke 'hansom cabs and other vehicles [finding] themselves on the footways' and the torturous route followed by a bemused 'pedestrian [who] could easily spend the evening looking for his house round the corner'. Analysing youthful feelings of isolation, he remembered '[slinking away] to one or other of the great railway termini with no more practical purpose than to see the hansoms lined up for the arrival of a long-distance express and so reassure myself that there really were limits to the be-sooted city, beyond which lay the fair rural shires and all the beauty of the woods and fields !' 'How utterly gruesome it was', Bonacina concluded, 'on such days of Stygian gloom to see the Victorian funerals, with their black steeds and craped mutes, stalking through the dismal streets.'[30] When he compared the metropolitan smoke fogs of the late nineteenth century with the infamous smog of 1952, he was unable to convince himself that the latter had been more intense or psychologically debilitating than intimidating episodes in the late Victorian period.

Counting environmental costs

In his famous *Sanitary Report* of 1842, Edwin Chadwick castigated local authorities for failing to introduce by-laws to punish habitual smoke polluters who had, in his view, simultaneously defiled the atmosphere and squandered scarce energy.[31] A major task was to find ways of applying established demographic cost-accounting procedures to the 'wilful' waste of domestic coal. Hints were provided in the fifth chapter of the *Sanitary Report* in which a Reverend G. Lewis noted that, in his native Dundee, 'fully one-half of the cases of fever occur in the prime of life when men are most useful either to their families or society'. Lewis went on to state that, over a period of seven years, 5,000 adults in the city had fallen ill with fever. Working on the assumption that an attack of the disease forced a typical labourer to stay off work for six weeks and that the average wage was 8s. a week, Lewis estimated the monetary loss attributable to fever at just over £12,500. Dispensary treatment – calculated at a pound a head – meant that an additional £5,000 should be added to the direct loss in wages. Attempting to estimate social costs associated with a further 5,000 cases among juvenile and adolescent dependants or semi-dependants, Lewis commented that 'as fever rarely attacks mere children, but chiefly those either in manhood or approaching manhood, we may estimate the loss of their labour at one-half of that of the adults ... and the expense of attendance and recovery as one half also'.[32] As for the 'cost of death', this was a complex as well as highly loaded matter. But, undaunted, Lewis concluded that:

> it seems a strange thing to set about estimating the money value of that which money did not give, and cannot restore when taken away: yet as there are those who understand better a profit and loss account than the arguments of religion and humanity, we shall attempt to estimate the [costs of] deaths by fever.[33]

Two years after the publication of the *Sanitary Report* the influential Commission into the State of Large Towns and Populous Districts concluded that 'solar light' was vital to the well-being of the urban working-class and that any depletion of so essential an element would lead to a deterioration in levels of vitality, health and income. As a result of reduced resistance, fever would flourish and prevent ever larger numbers of working people from following their 'ordinary occupations'. Family income would be eroded as a result of substantial amounts expended on 'procuring the assistance of those who have to attend [the sick] in illness'. 'Solar deficit' would also make heavy demands on funds that the 'benevolent subscribe to fever hospitals and other institutions'.[34] Precipitating enervation and depression, adverse atmospheric conditions could be expected to compromise national labour power. Atmospheric deterioration might even prove as pernicious as fever. When questioned by the Commission, Thomas Cubitt noted that working people were 'less willing to have expensive paper-hanging, and nice painting, and nice upholstery, because everything gets so black in London'.[35] William Guy estimated that, in London as a whole, an extra half a million pounds a year would need to be spent to undo the damage inflicted by atmospheric pollution.[36] The Marquess of Landsdowne claimed that metropolitan 'smoke so affected the clothing of the working classes that it was computed that every mechanic paid at least five times the amount of the original cost of his shirt for the number of washings rendered necessary'.[37]

In the early 1850s Chadwick's personal physician, Neil Arnott, the patentee of a 'smoke-consuming and fuel-saving fire-place', developed a 'weak calculus' which suggested that smoke fogs added to the 'cost of washing the clothes of inhabitants of London . . . by two millions and a half sterling a year'. Voicing proto-entropic anxiety, Arnott insisted that to 'consume coal wastefully and unnecessarily . . . is not merely improvidence but . . . a serious crime committed against future generations'.[38] These comments were made in a cultural environment in which it was widely believed that heat and energy, on which every advanced urban civilization depended, were being immorally squandered: within a decade, the publication of W.S. Jevons's *The Coal Question* would trigger a national debate about how to cut back on the consumption of domestic coal and avoid regression to arctic and primitive conditions of life.[39]

Glossing Arnott's estimates, Chadwick calculated that the annual metropolitan 'washing bill' had soared, by the mid-1850s, to the indefensible figure of £5 m. Reshaping a discourse that had thus far been almost wholly directed at the putatively improvident and intemperate working-class, Chadwick concluded that the metropolitan middle-classes – his natural constituency – were now forced to spend between a twelfth and a thirteenth of their annual per capita income on the washing and repeated rewashing of clothes.[40]

When atmospheric conditions deteriorated yet further in the early 1870s a group of meteorologists and social reformers – the most influential of whom was F.A.R. (Rollo) Russell – set out to estimate the social costs of metropolitan smoke fog. The son of the great Lord John and co-guardian of the young Bertrand Russell and his brother Frank at Pembroke Lodge in Richmond Park, Russell was educated at Christ Church, Oxford. He joined the Foreign Office but, as a result of extreme timidity and exceptionally poor eye-sight, rapidly withdrew from public employment. Back at Pembroke Lodge, Russell devoted himself to a wide range of meteorological and atmospheric studies. A passionate believer in the socially and morally reviving potential of rural life, he became increasingly disturbed by the impact of smoke fog on the health of the capital. In 1880 Russell published the first and most controversial of a series of books and pamphlets on atmospheric pollution. A best-seller, his *London Fog* mirrored increasingly pessimistic metropolitan attitudes towards the recurring fog phenomenon; stimulated a wide-ranging newspaper debate; and played a crucial role in establishing the capital's first anti-smoke pressure-group, the National Smoke Abatement Institution.

During the next 25 years Russell wrote extensively on a wide range of topics – the atmospheric determinants of epidemic disease, rural regeneration, and the history of the Liberal Party – but remained deeply committed to cataloguing and publicizing the socially, economically and medically deleterious impact of London fog.[41] In terms of epidemiological effects, Russell worked on the assumption that every case of atmospherically-related illness involved:

a loss of ten days, work [and that this gave] 70,000,000 days' work lost which might have been preserved. If half the number of cases are in adults earning 2s. a day, it appears that the loss to the nation in work and work alone that might be saved amounts to £3,500,000 a year.[42]

He enumerated no fewer than 25 variables, including the (now mandatory) 'extra washing', 'destruction of mortar', 'extra chimney sweeping', 'fuel burnt owing to want of sunshine caused by smoke', 'children kept from school' and 'damage to plants and natural life'. Drawing on sources and methodologies similar to those developed by Chadwick and Arnott, he arrived at a final estimate which confirmed Chadwick's earlier and probably at that time over-stated figure. This sum rapidly attained quasi-official status.[43] That each selected variable repeatedly suggested others, logically and sequentially inseparable from it, demonstrated the extent to which late nineteenth century London fog had insinuated itself into every cranny of social, economic and cultural life.

Russell's approach had inspired other attempts to calculate the costs of recurrent atmospheric pollution in the capital. In 1885 W. T. Makins, governor of the Gas, Light and Coke Company, argued that a recent spell of foggy weather had cost the public an extra £5,250 for gas, a sum that they could ill afford.[44] Making the case for legislative control before a select committee in 1887, Ernest Hart, editor of the *British Medical Journal* and pioneering anti-smoke activist, argued that his proposed measure would lead to:

a saving to the person in not having his furniture and curtains spoilt: in not having his books destroyed: and in not having the front of his house destroyed. If you come to put cost against saving there is no doubt the expenditure is as nothing compared to the economy.[45]

The 'actual cost in pounds, shillings and pence', Hart continued, 'can be shown to be at least £4 or £5 million a year in the metropolis'.[46] Two years later a popular meteorological periodical attempted to compute the costs of a typical smoke fog in the capital. Having noted extra payments of £3,000 that had been paid to

the Gas, Light and Coke Company, the journal claimed that it was
also necessary to incorporate:

> payments to other companies: extra electric lighting, lamps
> etc., the cost of damaged goods, damaged vehicles, damaged
> health, and surely for London alone we may put the cost of one
> day's fog at from £6,000 to £10,000. And though that were the
> worst, we have had quite twenty bad ones – take each of these
> as only half as bad, and we get the total damage of from
> £60,000 to £100,000, irrespective of the enormous amount of
> money taken out of the country by those who do not come to
> visit us during our foggy season.[47]

These cost-accounting exercises focused intensively on the needs of
the middle and respectable working-classes and paid little attention
to the daily lives of the London poor, a point well illustrated by
Viscount Midleton in 1891 when he told the House of Lords that:

> many of the working classes are prevented from following their
> daily occupations when a dense fog comes on: many more of
> them have to carry on their work under circumstances which are
> not only difficult but absolutely dangerous to themselves: and
> many more, again, who have not the advantage of medical
> treatment and proper nourishment, suffer terribly from the
> after effects of being exposed for days and weeks together
> during such weather as we have had lately to a tainted
> atmosphere which undermines their health and prevents them
> altogether from earning their living ...[48]

But the great majority of reformers continued to be preoccupied
with the health and well-being of the metropolitan professional,
governmental and scientific elites and the environmental, residential
and imperial integrity of the areas in which they lived. This was
particularly well demonstrated by prevailing attitudes towards
London's parks and gardens. In 1892 the Director of the Royal
Gardens at Kew lamented that fog deposits were destroying shrubs

and trees.[49] Throughout the capital the plane tree had become 'the past's theme, poor fellow! He cannot find any other trees in London to sing about. The freshest of flowers in the parks are jaded in a day; the very grass cannot grow green; it is in perpetual mourning.'[50] The gardens of the 'better class' had become no more than 'eyesores of limp grass, smutty paths and enfeebled privets and acubas'.[51] According to commentators like Ernest Hart, the lead would now have to be taken by the upper-middle classes who should be encouraged to persuade artisans to reduce consumption of the domestic fuel which constituted the principal cause of intolerable levels of atmospheric pollution during winter and early spring. Such an example would gradually wean the working-classes away from the attractions of the domestic grate and stimulate increased consumption of gas.[52]

New patterns of fog-associated disease

Lacking access to reliable information on city-wide patterns of cause-specific mortality, medical men in early nineteenth century London were nevertheless convinced that there were strong connections between cold and foggy weather and an increase in the incidence of debilitating and potentially fatal respiratory disease. Reviewing his case-book for January 1794 William Bent recorded that air in the capital had been 'very unfit for respiration': large numbers of his patients had complained of pain in the chest which had frequently been 'accompanied with a dry cough ... with children in particular this degenerated into [w]hooping cough, which became very universal'.[53] Describing similar conditions in the autumn of 1796 Robert Willan noted the prevalence of 'coughs and consumption' but argued that such illnesses were produced 'independently of the variations in temperature, or of the smoky, clogged atmosphere of London'.[54] Thomas Bateman, by contrast, remained convinced that the 'influence of fogs' could be decisive. Writing about exceptionally polluted conditions in the capital during the winter of 1809–10, he stated that 'the occurrence of frost invariably multiplies the number of pulmonary disorders; but when it is conjoined with thick fogs, it is doubly pernicious, from the greater rapidity with which the atmosphere, thus loaded, abstracts the heat of the body'.[55]

Until the middle of the nineteenth century there was a consensus that those susceptible to respiratory problems – and particularly asthma – would deteriorate, and might even have their health irreparably damaged, if they spent too much time out of doors during severe smoke fogs.[56] A pessimistic minority went further and argued that 'the presence of soot particles' led to 'black mucus [being] expectorated from the lungs during a November fog ... peculiar to London'.[57] In general, however, medical men and public health activists agreed with Andrew Ure when he informed a select committee investigating legislative means of reducing levels of metropolitan pollution that fog 'oppresses people of weak lungs. Robust people may resist those impressions longer, but the weakly are very sensible to it, particularly when the smoke will not rise, in cold weather'.[58]

By mid-century public health specialists and environmental reformers were lending their support to a different and more generalized set of arguments. According to this view, numerous yellow smoke fogs had already created an environment in which working-class members of the metropolitan population were becoming stunted and incapable of reproducing a strong and healthy stock. According to this interpretation, the inhabitants of the eastern and central districts had for too long been:

> shut up within close apartments, removed from the direct rays of the sun, hidden from the sight of the blue sky and the white clouds, and immersed beneath a canopy of smoke and lofty buildings ... how [would it be] possible for the functions of life to develop themselves at large, with their natural energy, and in their due proportions? It is evidently impossible; intra- and extra-uterine vitality are equally arrested and deformed; the blood loses its full measure of oxygen, and is deprived of the ruby tint, so characteristic of health and vigour; the limbs are small, the joints large, the chest narrow, the forehead hydrocephalic, the teeth irregular, the hair lank, the mind morbidly keen, and the passions perverted or depraved.[59]

Not only had working-class Londoners been deprived of 'natural solar health' during the fog season: tainted air seeping into their houses and tenements had compelled them to keep their windows shut. As a consequence, 'the close smell of food, and dress, and human exhalation, and, above all, the gases which rush into the warmed home from every drain and dustheap upon the premises' either led to outbreaks of fever or − 'quite literally' − to 'suffocation'.[60] Such representations were influenced by venerable stereotypes of the urban primitive or savage, a category that had developed out of mid-eighteenth century conceptions of racial hierarchies within and between cultures, the stages of development postulated by classical economic theory and the new proto-anthropology of the early nineteenth century. These images rapidly gained currency among the first generation of metropolitan sanitary reformers, and, following the revolution in evolutionary thinking, reemerged in scientistic social Darwinistic form as a means of comprehending, interpreting and castigating the behaviour of the urban poor.[61]

Racialized conceptions of this kind were intimately linked to the idea that a depleted internal economy of air within the individual dwelling might precipitate a wide range of potentially fatal conditions, ranging from a low count of red corpuscles to debility or fully fledged fever. When combined with high levels of external atmospheric pollution, lack of internal ventilation would prove deadly. As, from the early 1870s onwards, atmospheric conditions deteriorated, meteorologists, sanitary reformers and cultural critics embraced overtly class-inflected variants of degenerationist discourses which diverted attention away from explicitly causal connexions between high levels of smoke fog and an increase in mortality from respiratory disease. Viewed from this catastrophist perspective, the capital − as well as urban life as a whole − might already be atmospherically doomed.

Between the 1840s and the early Edwardian period, then, sanitarian, racialized, degenerationist and anti-urban discourses dominated debate in relation to the severity of London's smoke fog problem. But from the early 1870s changes in procedures at the General Registry Office began to produce findings which demonstrated that age- and cause-specific death rates associated with atmospheric pollution in the capital might be even higher than the 'excess mortality' experienced during the metropolitan cholera epidemics of 1848–9, 1854–5 and 1866. These innovations served to reinforce intensely pessimistic perceptions of the depth and intensity of the fog crisis.

During the two generations between the 1840s and the early Edwardian period atmospheric and ventilationist theories of this kind were ever more heavily influenced by anti-urbanism. Cities, it was argued, could not be demographically self-sufficient: ever larger numbers of rural immigrants were therefore needed – and were in fact being successfully recruited – to make good the deficit attributable to 'residual' elements who, as a result of inherited weakness and morally disreputable life-style, were failing to sustain their genealogical 'line' for more than three generations.[62] Both in the case of native city-dwellers and recent arrivals from the countryside, metropolitan fog was said to accelerate this process.

Dragging down vitality, making depressing housing and living conditions more enervating, a dark and murky climate tempted the working-class – even more so the residuum – to seek out apparently spirit-reviving but in fact libidinously immoral relief. Whenever there was incessant fog, it was much easier to lose sense of self and social responsibility, with the result, again, that alcohol might become more tempting than during more favourable climatic conditions.[63] Finally, fog, through the visual and aural isolation of individuals and groups, separated and segregated the classes at precisely that moment at which urban moral fragmentation and decline demanded ever more intensive intermingling, so that example might be transmitted to those who might otherwise be morally lost.[64]

Young female immigrants, born and bred in supposedly idyllic village communities, had long been believed to be more vulnerable to the temptations of urban sin than men. Alleged to be disillusioned by endless and futile rounds of washdays forced on them by London murk, such individuals were said to become indifferent to domestic and personal hygiene and then to descend into inertia and depression.

The next – inevitable – step would be to seek out the moralist's 'bright and cheerful light' which would eventually lure them into irresponsibility, intemperance and vice.[65] In terms of escape, sick or debilitated members of the social elite were, of course, free to leave the capital whenever they wished: and many did, heading either for the countryside or southern Europe.[66] But working people had no option but to stay where they were, as near-total darkness and atmospheric impurity intermittently lowered spirits, undermined constitutions and fostered inbred and hereditarily communicable debility. It was only a short step from a formulation of this kind to the gloomy prognostication that the London fog was both cause and frightening symbol of full-scale urban decline.

By the time that the capital had become engulfed in its late nineteenth century atmospheric crisis, explicitly medical modes of analysis had been largely superseded by post-sanitarian, degenerationist interpretation. Surveying St Giles, Douglas Galton doubted whether it would ever be possible for fully-formed human beings to emerge from such 'foul, gloomy dwellings, in to which it is impossible that a ray of sunshine or pure air can ever penetrate'.[67] Adopting the obsessively anti-urban perspective that would dominate his later writings, Rollo Russell hypothesized that the origins of metropolitan moral evil could be traced back to the moment at which contact had been lost with the 'clear azure above'.[68] In the eyes of the metropolitan middle-class and professional and scientific elites, social, biological, meteorological and medical processes had become inextricably intertwined.[69] Ernest Hart lamented that 'when you have, as we have in London now, the rays of light continuously obstructed, you have all the processes of life continually lowered'.[70]

Doom of a great city?

At an extreme – in William Delisle Hay's sensationalist *Doom of the Great City* – the London smoke fog came to symbolize the intense social, economic and political insecurities of the late Victorian city. Converting the real fog of February 1880 into a suffocating and 'strangulating killer smog', Hay chronicled a saga of misapplied wealth, moral and social perversion and sexual excess. Even more obsessively and misogynistically than most other contemporaries, he projected the squalor of the capital on to the 'garish' and 'painted' wives, mistresses and courtesans of the 'top ten thousand'. 'London', Hay's narrator ruminates, 'was foul and rotten to the very base, and steeped in sin of every imaginable variety': it was impossible to 'contemplate the Londoners of those days without a feeling of disgust and loathing springing up from within you'.[71] No less pernicious had been the 'dictatorship of fashion' whereby 'aestheticism' had served as a 'cloak for the higher flights of sin'. Little wonder that, in this ethical climate, 'prostitution [had] flourished so abundantly in London as scarcely to be looked upon as a vice at all, except by the most rigorous': or that, under cover of darkness and fog, 'garotters, burglars, and all the guilds of open crime revelled in contented impurity'.[72]

The day before Hay's 'normal' metropolitan fog is transformed into a smog that will 'kill thousands', the narrator visits the home of an elite professional family living in the semi-rural comfort of Dulwich. This is the privileged social and topographical vantage-point from which, early the next morning, he glimpses the deadly 'killer cloud' lower itself over the central city districts. As half-stifled commuters stumble back from the railway station, Hay, following the dictates of a pre-determined narrative, thrusts his protagonist once more back into the centre of the 'doomed city' in an attempt to save a beloved mother and sister. 'I must', he says, 'go back to the very heart and home of Horror itself'.[73] All this prepares the way for the mounting of a series of quasi-cinematic *natures mortes*, detailing, in luridly melodramatic tonality, the suffocation of the London elite. Resplendently groomed horses sprawl, half-asphxyiated, across Mayfair's 'streets of pleasure': coachmen, seemingly alive, wait, stiff-backed and lifeless, outside great West End houses: at Buckingham Palace *rigor mortis* holds a guardsman to attention in a caricature of ceremonialism.

A theatre audience waits, 'strangulated', in gorgeous evening finery, for a curtain that will never rise, while 'behind [it] stretch[ed] the "pit" filled with its crowd of commoner folk, mingled and inextricably involved in a chaos of heads and limbs and bodies, writhed and knotted together into one great mass of dead men, dead women, and dead children, too'.[74] The destruction of a ruling class, which had knowingly reneged on its ordained duty towards its social inferiors, is ghoulishly catalogued. Diamonds glitter in the gutter: the bejewelled hand of an aristocratic pleasure-seeker reaches out across a table in a crowded restaurant as her companion slides, half-dead, to the floor.

The fate of the working-class, by contrast, is assumed rather than narrated or cumulatively visualized: in this sense, Hay implies, the everyday, chronic, 'non-strangulating' fog has already inexorably eroded both communal vitality and the biological will to survive. A kind of pity there certainly is, but it is expressed in the moralized and tragi-sentimental tone that characterized nearly all late Victorian debate of decline and putative demographic collapse. We need hardly add that the narrator's mother and sister do indeed perish, 'strangled' in the sitting-room of their 'modest' cottage. A similar fate awaits 'miserable [children] in the gutter, two poor little ragged urchins, barefooted, filthy, half-naked outcasts of the streets, their meagre limbs cuddled round each other in a last embrace, their poor parched faces pressed together in a last embrace and upturned to heaven. To them, perhaps, death had been but release from life.'[75]

Can the darkness lift?

Like Dickens before them, novelists and poets from every level of the literary hierarchy appropriated the London fog as a potent symbol of rediscovered metropolitan poverty and environmental deprivation. In so doing, they probed an even more sombre darkness at the heart of the metropolitan and imperial projects.[76] Gissing and Conrad worked this seam.[77] So, also, did Richard Jefferies, James Thomson and Conan Doyle.[78] Jefferies' *After London* depicts a city-scape which, in the aftermath of an obscure but devastating natural (or man-made?) calamity, is returned to a state of nature. This narrative precisely mirrored the preoccupations and proposed panaceas of urban and social reformers convinced that the capital must now make a final attempt to escape from its atmospheric fate. By the early 1890s, then, potential solutions to the objective environmental problem itself – the incidence and intensity of the London smoke fogs – had been submerged beneath a babble of degenerationist voices obsessed, like Hay's, with something akin to global despair. Many of those involved in the debate now proposed radical rural and agrarian solutions.

At an extreme, these constituted nothing less than an attempt to wish the capital – and all its works – out of existence. Rollo Russell, who had first alerted influential sectors of public opinion to the necessity of confronting atmospheric pollution in the aftermath of the crises of 1873 and 1880, now championed the creation of a new moral order in which the sun would renovate human health and itself become a symbol of god's immanence. Restored communal vitality would be underwritten by scientific innovation, with the latter being placed in the service of divine purpose.[79] By 1905, with metropolitan fog smoke less menacing, Rollo Russell was still insisting that the 'populations of the central parts of our big towns [will] decline and perish unless continually recruited from the country. And thousands are ever flocking from country to town. Only by a return to the country, or by great improvements in the conditions of urban life, can the nation maintain its prosperity.'[80]

Although sanitarian, ventilationist and degenerationist discourses decisively shaped the cultural framing of London's smoke fogs between the 1840s and the early twentieth century, changes in demographic and epidemiological perspectives also played an important role. During the 1870s official attention continued to be predominantly focused on environmentally-transmitted infections – the so-called 'zymotic' group. Nevertheless, a growing body of writing now focused on the etiology and possible interractions between tuberculosis, pneumonia, bronchitis, whooping-cough and general respiratory disease.[81] As we have seen, following the great fog of 1873, the General Registry Office confirmed the existence of a similar kind of excess mortality to that which had been experienced in the capital during each of the mid-century cholera epidemics.[82]

But this additional death-toll might be no more than the tip of an iceberg. As the ever-vigilant Rollo Russell had speculated in 1880:

> the death-rate during a few days of dense fog palpably mounts to an extraordinary degree, but every year we have a large number of ordinary London fogs of less density which, lasting as they commonly do only one or two days ... fail to affect the death-rate sufficiently to be noted ...[83]

Despite this weakness, statistical analysis had nevertheless finally confirmed what medical opinion and commonsense had long assumed – that the elderly and the very young were greatly more vulnerable to illness or death during densely foggy weather than all other age-groups. But the precise scale of mortality and morbidity from specific forms of respiratory disease, and the extent to which their incidence was directly or indirectly related to metropolitan smoke fog, would remain an elusive field of inquiry.[84]

Between 1873 and the early 1890s London was repeatedly afflicted by severe episodes of fog which paralyzed social and economic life, precipitated high levels of excess mortality and gave rise to deeply pessimistic attitudes towards urban and 'cosmic' existence. Between 1893 and 1903, however, the annual number of episodes significantly declined.[85] By the end of the century the *Lancet* was reporting that 'though there was gloom, artificial light was not resorted to on anything like the scale of old when day was night. The air of London has been clearer lately and the densely smoking chimney appears to be the exception rather than the rule among the myriad that abound.'[86] Causal processes were unclear but, in 1901, a veteran anti-fog campaigner commented that a 'great difference has taken place in the atmosphere ... we had more than the normal number of misty days, but not one of those black fogs with which we are annually plagued during the winter'.[87] In 1906 the Registrar-General reported that in 'Westminster there were only 16 days on which fog was recorded, less than one third of the normal frequency, the smallest numbers in previous years being 13 in 1900 and 26 in 1903'.[88]

In 1908 'one of the marked features of the year was the almost entire absence of any great fogs over the land', a pattern which was repeated in 1910.[89] By the beginning of World War I, the *British Medical Journal* was confidently reporting that 'the present generation happily knows little of the "London particulars" which used to afflict the dwellers in the metropolis thirty years ago'.[90] But the fogs returned. Conditions were periodically severe during the inter-war years. Then in 1948 and even more ferociously in 1952 London found itself assailed by death-dealing smog.[91] Once again newspapers and periodicals – abetted by radio, newsreels and embryonic television – relayed images of cosmic doom. Yet now, increasingly sophisticated analysis at the level of cause- and age-specific mortality more accurately pinpointed the numbers of elderly inhabitants who had perished from respiratory and heart disease.

Eighty years earlier, according to Simon Szreter, 'social Darwinism [had] swept through English bourgeois society and conquered, at least temporarily, many of its most influential social commentators, social scientists and important figures in the biodmedical sciences'. Moreover, 'a simplistically socialized Darwinism, with its maxim of survival of the fittest':

> [had undermined] the rationale for a public health policy by implying that resources invested in ... measures were a misguided waste, merely prolonging the lives of nature's weaklings. It could be argued that measures to reduce the infant and child mortality of the 'residuum' ... would merely be cancelled-out in greater morbidity and mortality rates at higher ages, as these unviable individuals hopelessly struggled to survive, clogging up the nation's labour market with enfeebled and inefficient 'stocks'.[92]

This chapter has pointed to significant continuities between sanitarian and ventilationist responses to the increasing severity of smoke fog in the capital in the 1840s and 1850s and predominantly social Darwinistic and degenerationist interpretations during the final thirty years of the century. Drawing on cost-accounting approaches which had attempted to place a monetary value on mortality and morbidity from fever, mid-century reformers became convinced that depleted solar resources had already heightened the probability that environmentally impoverished Londoners would experience a deterioration in health and produce large numbers of debilitated offspring. Importing elements of miasmatic theory into this proto-degenerationist scenario, they contended that atmospheric deprivation precipitated by smoke fog would be further exacerbated by counter-productive internal ventilatory arrangements that might in the longer term 'strangle' all those compelled to live in close and airless conditions. This florid and seemingly indefinitely flexible discourse survived fundamentally unchanged until the Edwardian period – in 1902 it could still be claimed that:

> a curious conglomeration of sand, salt, soot, cotton fibres, vegetable debris, bacteria and their spores, diatoms, monads, infusoria, pollen of flower and grasses, pulverised straw, and epithetical scales from the skin, when inspissated, as it is in towns, assists in the production of a low state of health and constitutional debility, especially amongst children, and [when combined with fog] ... conduces to a wide spread mortality.[93]

When, between the 1870s and the mid-1890s, the patina of the London fog ominously changed from dirty yellow to gritty black, elite reactions became even more pessimistic. Miasmatically-based sanitarianism continued to be espoused by a minority of medical men and environmental reformers, but could no longer command the support that it had possessed between the mid-1840s and the 1860s. Now, however, a novel and even more adaptable resource – social Darwinism – made itself available. Manipulated literally and metaphorically, this most persuasive of ideologies rhetorically completed a narrative initiated in the 1840s. Unremitting fog in late nineteenth century London would 'suffocate' the population of the inner districts, while at the same time serving as a symbol of irremediable urban, biological and national decline. The opportunity for a solution – whether technological, legislative, economic or social – had been squandered. Only a genuinely radical programme, based on rural regeneration and a strengthening of metropolitan charitable and religious bonds, would be capable of dragging the doomed city back from the brink.

In the early Edwardian period, when anti-metropolitan discourses of this kind reached their zenith, London's smoke fog suddenly became less threatening. The respite was widely welcomed. But there would be no return to the white and 'country-like' episodes experienced during 'normal' years in the late eighteenth and early nineteenth centuries. Climatically, epidemiologically and ideologically, the great London fogs had done their work.

CHAPTER 8

UNENDING DEBATE: TOWN, COUNTRY AND THE CONSTRUCTION OF THE RURAL IN ENGLAND, 1870–2000

Against the urban grain

The green belt continues to retain its potency as a symbol of a deep gulf between town and country in modern and contemporary Britain, a buffer pointing to imbedded and radically divergent conceptions of differences between the rural and urban spheres.[1] Its very existence underlines the fact that, in the twentieth century and in our own times, the assumed integrity of village life and mores have counted for significantly more than celebration of regional or civic values and culture. The belt was originally intended to fence off agricultural land bordering the metropolitan perimeter from ever more rapid, and as many contemporaries termed it, octopus-like extra-urban expansion.[2] Reaching back to the initiatives of the London County Council and the Campaign for the Preservation (later Protection) of Rural England in the early 1930s, the belt was strengthened by the post-war Greater London Plan, masterminded by the extraordinarily influential planning supremo, Patrick Abercrombie.[3]

In 1955 and again in 1971 it was finally and formally installed as an instrument of central and local bureaucratic control.[4] The ground had been prepared in two phases, between the 1870s and the beginning of World War I, and between 1918 and the resumption of hostilities in 1939. Thereafter, the period of reconstruction between the mid-1940s and the late 1950s witnessed increased commitment on the part of government and a now mature planning bureaucracy to the idea that one or another variant of an essential rural England must be insulated against urban and suburban development.[5] This orthodoxy remained dominant for 40 years. Only in the recent past, with complex questions being asked about changing relationships between town, suburbia and countryside has there been a weakening of the idea that rural England must remain indefinitely sacrosanct.[6]

During the 1990s and on into the beginning of the new century, this reevaluation gave rise to the founding of the Countryside Alliance. The Alliance capitalized on a wide range of rural discontent, including closure of village primary schools, banks and post offices, the adverse impact of the Common Agricultural Policy on farmers attempting to make a living from small acreages, the trimming or eradication of rail and bus services and governmental commitment to the control or abolition of hunting and coursing.[7] The Alliance has revived the venerable idea that modern Britain is dominated by London, and administered predominantly in the interests of the inhabitants of London and other great conurbations. Between the 1870s and 1945, and earlier, anti-urbanism and anti-metropolitanism played a prominent role in British, and even more so in English, cultural life. Since the medieval period the precocious demographic and spatial growth of the capital had engendered widespread apprehension and hostility. This generated elite and popular literary traditions associating London with corruption, environmental and moral pollution and disdain for the assumed ignorance of the inhabitants of smaller towns and villages.[8]

During the 130 years with which this chapter is concerned, diffuse consensus was transformed into a mature anti-urban, anti-metropolitan discourse articulated by organizations such as the Kyrle Society, the Royal Society for the Protection of Birds, the Society for Saving the Natural Beauty of the Lake District, the

Council for the Preservation of Rural England, and later and in our own times, the National Trust and English Heritage. Associated literary lineages have been long and distinguished, running from Chaucer to Spencer, from Shakespeare and Jonson to Milton's *Comus*, and in the eighteenth and nineteenth centuries, from Gay, Goldsmith, Clare and Blake to the pioneering laureate-cum- proto-ecologist, William Wordsworth.[9] Thereafter, representative figures included Ruskin and Morris, Gissing, Conrad, Woolf, Eliot, Lawrence and Forster. In their different ways, these thinkers and writers massively idealized the rural sphere, and castigated urban-industrialism as a progenitor of soulless modernity and interpersonal alienation. Simultaneously many writers and cultural critics excoriated the 'civilization of the machine'.[10]

Anti-urban and anti-metropolitan writers, particularly Gissing, Morris and Richard Jefferies, created rural utopias as a counter-weight to town-based addiction to mass production and mass consumption. Eliot, echoing ideas first articulated by Blake in his terrifying poem, 'London', and by Wordsworth in the seventh book of the *Prelude*, mordantly associated urban gigantism with literary analogues to Durkheimian anomie.[11] Among composers Elgar, Delius, Vaughn Williams, Finze, Ireland, Britten, and the early Tippett created soundscapes which reflected similar anti-urban preoccupations.[12] English painters from the pre-Raphaelites to Spencer, Grant, Nash and Sutherland remained at least partially in thrall to the rural idyll.[13]

Above all, however, it was London – and the condition of London – which obsessed anti-urbanists in the long period between the fifteenth and the mid-twentieth century. The premature demo-graphic expansion of the capital, its all-embracing incorporation of the super-wealthy and the abjectly poor, and its seemingly illimitable spatial ambition, promised to undermine the sacred project of civilizing the city. The capital boasted a population of a quarter of a million at the beginning of the seventeenth century, three times that number a century later, a million a century after that, 2.5 million in 1850, 4.5 million in the 1880s and no fewer than seven million at the end of World War I.[14]

From the 1870s onwards the populations of the largest of the metropolitan townships, or registration districts, spiraled upwards to between 150,000 and 300,000. Had they possessed independent urban status, places like St Pancras, Marylebone, Wandsworth, Camberwell and Hammersmith, would have occupied an impressive position in the league tables assiduously compiled by mid- and late Victorian and Edwardian social statisticians and reformers.[15] Several substantial 'new industrial districts' in the midlands and north – Nottingham, Leicester, Derby, Bolton and Blackburn – were significantly smaller than the largest of the London suburbs, a point lost on commentators more concerned with the alleged failure of the capital to modernize and democratize its supposedly medieval governmental system than with comparative urban demographics.[16] For their part, most Londoners appeared to know and care little about life in urban-industrial Britain.

Nevertheless, and despite the existence of deeply ingrained anti-metropolitanism in places like Birmingham, Manchester and Leeds, the sheer longevity and scale of the capital ensured that the capital became synonymous with cities and the ills of cities in general. The East End symbolized hopeless poverty, and the metropolitan suburbs provided a paradigm for the way in which major centres of population preyed upon and appropriated hitherto administratively independent extra-urban communities. London, a giant among giants, was perceived as a constant threat to the spatial integrity of small towns and villages lying just outside what would later come to be designated the greater metropolitan region. Little wonder, then, that social and cultural critics, and, later, planners and environmentalists concentrated on the problems of the London-dominated south, rather than the midlands and north, the arable English heartland rather than Scotland, Ireland or Wales. Together with a cluster of organizations concerned with the protection of the Lake District, it was metropolitan intellectuals, bureaucrats and politicians who shaped rural preservationism in the later nineteenth and early twentieth centuries. In that sense, as in many other things, Anglocentric prevailed over larger British values and concerns.[17]

Imagined rural colonies

Urban reformers, disturbed by the overweening outward expansion of the capital, settled to a quite astonishing degree on a single, phantasmagoric solution – stabilization of metropolitan population through a recolonization of traditional village communities.[18] Theories of this kind were predicated on rejuvenation of rural trades, crafts and industries believed to have flourished before the onset of capitalistic farming in the post-medieval period. 'Reskilled' unemployed dockers would now enjoy healthier and happier lives in village and hamlet. Multiform social, economic and epidemiological problems associated with the inner city would be partially solved, and the quality of the national stock, central to intellectuals and reformers in thrall to the idea of urban degeneration and eugenics, significantly reduced.[19] Aggregate metropolitan population and movement from inner core to suburban periphery would be held steady, giving rise to a deceleration in the rate of suburban expansion, and capping 'colonizing' pressure on neighbouring extra-metropolitan communities.

This panacea, combining Ruskin's and Morris's rural utopianism with what would have amounted to semi-compulsory relocation policies, ignored what Karl Marx described as the real existing conditions of demand and supply in urban and rural labour markets. Its emergence and discursive dominance coincided with a period of agricultural recession. The idea of a nationwide 'great depression' between the early 1870s and mid-1890s has been banished from the literature. However, there is now agreement that regional and climatic factors, together with new and cheaper supplies of meat and cereals from Australasia and Canada, did indeed trigger extremely severe regional difficulties.[20] Moreover, the push and pull of internal migration had already reduced the proportion of the adult population able to derive a living from working on the land. Comprising nearly a fifth of the workforce in the 1850s, agricultural labourers accounted for slightly less than a tenth at the beginning of the twentieth century, a figure that would plunge downwards to little more than a fiftieth over the next 75 years. Little chance, then, of an East Ham docker finding a job in Thomas Hardy's depopulated Dorset or the broad acres of a Norfolk now registering significant levels of emigration to precisely those parts of the Empire – Canada and Australia – that had played a crucial role in increasing arable unemployment and under-employment.[21]

Florid rhetoric advocating rural regeneration and relocation of the metropolitan poor to the depths of the countryside appealed both to paternalistic conservatives and modernizing progressives.[22] By the final 30 years of the nineteenth century each of these groups had adopted an increasingly negative or ambivalent attitude towards the possibility of creating what would now be termed an ecologically and socially sustainable urban civilisation. A generation earlier, liberals had seen newly emerging self-governing cities as beacons of progress which would play a central historical role in the emancipation of the working-classes and the final destruction of 'feudalism'.[23] For its part, the landed interest depicted both London and new industrial towns in the midlands and north as inimical to health, happiness and morality. By the 1870s and 1880s both groups had experienced radical ideological and cultural fragmentation and reconstitution: each had been reshaped within the arenas of parliamentary, municipal and pressure-group politics. However, many of those still definable as liberals or progressives now perceived the city, industrialization and urban-industrialism as inadequate to the tasks of reducing economic scarcity, securing individual happiness and creating the good society. For their part, paternalist conservatives claimed that their original doubts about the moral defensibility and spatial viability of the city and manufacturing industry had been well-founded.

At the same time, history and the professionalization of history as an academic discipline, reinforced doubts about the past achievements and future potential of a machine-dominated society. There had, of course, been profoundly pessimistic and critical voices in the early and mid-nineteenth century. Then in 1881–2 Arnold Toynbee radically and authoritatively modified over-sanguine views of the seismic shift towards an industrial culture.[24] This interpretation shaped English social, though not economic, history throughout the Edwardian and interwar eras and beyond. John and Barbara

Hammond gained a massive academic and non-academic readership for their studies of town and village labourers during the early phases of industrialization.[25] G.M. Trevelyan's expansive social history, written for a general audience, abounds with references to the cruelty, profiteering and pollution of factory culture, and massively idealizes conditions of life in preindustrial society.[26] This pessimistic *mentalite* lay at the heart of E.P. Thompson's classic *The Making of the English Working Class*, published in 1963, and sustained itself in residual form until the demise of institutional and academic Marxism in the late 1980s.[27]

The Hammonds' catastrophist interpretation was echoed by inter-war intellectuals, rural preservationists and planners. However, it was now also widely believed that knowledge of and exposure to the beauties of nature might do something to bind up the wounds of an urban working-class, said to have been grievously harmed by exposure to the miseries of urban-industrialism. This analysis was applied both to the period of the industrial revolution and to the collapse of the primary-producing manufacturing sector in the 1930s. Thinkers as influential and culturally diverse as Trevelyan – co-founder of the Council for the Preservation of Rural England as well as eminent historian – Patrick Abercrombie, J.M. Keynes and E.M. Forster subscribed to one or another variant of this view.[28]

At an extreme, D.H. Lawrence insisted on nothing less than an absolute renunciation of the city and all its works – urban-industrialism, the machine, mass consumption and mass entertainment.[29] Trevelyan contended that a solution might lie in controlled access to nature. According to this schema, the ills of urban-industrialism would gradually be corrected through popular rambling, youth hostelling and climbing.[30] Patrick Abercrombie adopted a different position, and one which would later underpin dominant values informing post-war reconstruction. Arguing that it might not be possible to undo the miseries of urban-industrialism by mass exposure to nature *in situ*, he urged that the countryside and countryside values must themselves be imported into the city. Were every town-dweller to be given an opportunity creatively to enjoy *rus in urbe*, while at the same time learning about and being educated in the customs, codes and responsibilities of the wild, he or she would become a physically, culturally and morally improved individual.[31] (The values of the early twentieth century garden city movement clearly and powerfully underscored Abercrombie's vision.[32]) There need be no contradiction between preserving rural values, securing enhanced access to the wilds, or to nature in the city, rebuilding and beautifying urban centres besmirched by dilapidated factory and slum, and championing one or another form of architectural modernism.[33] Each of these positions may be traced back to the perceived metropolitan crisis of the late nineteenth century. Yet, and this point cannot be too strongly emphasized, London was in reality the *least* classically industrial of the great cities of Britain. However, its status as massive and long-established super-metropolis ensured that it became a symbol and paradigm to which consensually negative attitudes towards urbanism, industrialism and urban-industrialism were unthinkingly, routinely and irrationally attached.

The pro-rural, anti-urban, anti-metropolitan discourses which flourished in Britain between the 1870s and 1945 and beyond was also rooted in and reinforced by differential response to world war and total war. The period between 1918 and 1939 witnessed an outpouring of literature which lamented national and familial loss or sought to create a compensatory arcadian moral universe. This included writings as diverse as Ford Madox Ford *Parade's End*; P.G. Wodehouse's massively popular evocations of a comically dysfunctional aristocratic and semi-aristocratic rural order; Hugh Walpole's popular recreations of a quasi-historical Lake District; Stanley Baldwin's ruminations on what constituted the 'real', ineradicable heart of England. Each was symptomatic of a cultural mood designed to eradicate memories of the Somme and return to an imagined Edwardian idyll.[34]

The impact of World War II was different. There was no lack of writing expressing a yearning for a rural – aristocratic, hierarchical and 'feudal' – past. Evelyn Waugh's *Brideshead Revisited* and Sword of Honour trilogy explore precisely this terrain.[35] The predominantly rurally rooted fiction of L.P. Hartley is located in a similar though

more worldly cultural milieu, while the extraordinarily popular
H.E. Bates and Laurie Lee luxuriated in unabashed rural nostalgia.[36]
In general, however, World War II generated a desire to forget rather
than reimagine, recover or reinvent. The economic disasters of the
1930s, the nadir of urban-industrialism, and failure on the part
of successive pre-war governments to frame policies which might
have reduced the trauma of mass unemployment, ensured that
the dominant mood tended to be forward-looking, disowning
rather than clinging to a mythological preindustrial past. Yet this
mood did little to weaken the attractions of anti-urban rural
preservationism. The election of a Labour government ensured that
social policies prepared during the middle years of the war were
rapidly implemented.[37] At the same time, planners had now come
of age and insisted that the blitz provided an inherently conservative
nation with an opportunity to undo what were now conventionally
assumed to be the environmental monstrosities of Victorian
industrialism.[38]

The polluted city would be cleansed by combining architectural
modernism with variants of *rus in urbe*. New towns and the
rebuilding of centres subjected to heavy bombing would deploy
zoning to validate the spatial coexistence of nature and – preferably
light – industry. At the same time planners experimented with city-
based schemes for suburbs underwritten by the values of hamlet and
village.[39] Social and architectural engineering were now thought to
be capable of reproducing elements of the rural within modernistic
architectural and residential settings.[40] Linked bodies of legislation
would be introduced to protect wildlife, wilderness and places of
natural beauty proximate to and far distant from the great city.[41]

Excluding and misrepresenting suburbia

The impact of a dominant discourse is enhanced by failure to engage
with a full range of empirical evidence. Commonsensical, natural,
a priori assumptions interact with linear logical structures to account
for no more than a limited spectrum of simplified social and
environmental variables to guarantee coherence, credibility and the

possibility for yet further simplification and popularization. Dominant discourses become even more persuasive if they can be readily absorbed by interest groups able to adapt central tenets to their own professional and social needs. Popularization and simplification also work in favour of effective dissemination throughout the social system as a whole.[42] As with election manifestos, so also with a dominant discourse, analysis and interpretation are less usefully concerned with evaluating policy solutions to convoluted social and economic problems than the ways in which complexity is rhetorically reduced to the familiar coinage of predictability.

Anglocentric, pro-rural preservationism in Britain between 1870 and 1945 gained in persuasiveness because it gave little detailed attention to the crucial issue of the material and social formation of an emergent national suburbia. As we have seen, perceived dilemmas associated with the octopus-like growth of the suburbs, particularly in London, generated wide-ranging comment. But throughout our period this debate was abstracted from its concrete economic, social and spatial contexts. Statistical generalization continues to be treacherous but in nearly every major urban centre between the 1860s and the 1940s and beyond suburban outpaced city-wide rates of population growth.[43] Commercialization of the urban core and the construction of central railway termini pushed those who could afford extra outgoings in terms of rent and travel to an inner suburban ring: a significant minority lacking the wherewithal to make such a move became – to use the standard Victorian euphemism – 'dishoused' and found themselves forced to endure levels of overcrowding as severe as those experienced in the 1840s.[44] Either that, or they had to find shelter on the unforgiving streets of the great city.

Every suburban area was different from its near-neighbour or from what might seem to be similar localities in other towns or cities.[45] In broadly schematic terms, outward movement from the inner core gave rise to successive residential rings. These accommodated finely differentiated sub-groups – better-off members of the working-class and the aristocracy of labour, non-manual employees in routine administrative jobs in the central business district, the lower middle-class, the middle class itself and what George Orwell famously termed the lower upper-middle class. At the periphery the affluent upper middle-class inhabited spacious detached villas. These elite members of the population lived in semi-rural splendour in communities retaining many of the characteristics of traditional village life but contained a significantly larger range and proportion of shopkeepers and tradesmen. In London, Hampstead and Highgate were the classic examples.[46]

The nationwide shift towards mass suburbanization, which began in London in the earliest years of the nineteenth century, and then replicated itself in Birmingham, Manchester, Leeds and smaller centres, would not have developed in the way it did in the absence of a regionally staggered upward shift in real income from the 1850s onwards.[47] Increased economic stability exerted a profound effect on residential and occupational change within the late Victorian city, and raised reality and expectation in terms of health, environment and amenity.[48] Later in the century, the development of mass transport systems, and particularly cheap fares, reinforced the suburbanizing process.[49] At the same time, those who remained behind at the inner core experienced a relative decline in health and amenity.[50] This was the era of the mass slum as well as mass suburbanization. Sometimes, as in the capital, the two spheres were organically linked to one another.[51]

Both in London and the great provincial centres communities bordering urban regions came gradually to accept that it would be in their own best interests to be formally incorporated into the great city. Thus in the late nineteenth century the villages of Chorlton, Withington and Didsbury allowed themselves to be administratively colonized by Manchester, thereby preparing the way for an even more massive suburban thrust deep into agricultural Cheshire during the inter-war era. In fact, it was during the 1920s and 1930s that residence in a terraced, semi-detached or detached property, far removed from the environmental *sturm und drang* of the urban core, became a dominant cultural as well as economic and residential norm.[52] At the same time, outsiders, inhabitants of the most deprived and least salubrious areas of cities, whose parents had lacked the wherewithal to escape to a respectable inner suburb, remained trapped in what had come by the 1880s to be known as the shamefully 'hidden' slums of London, Manchester, Leeds and Birmingham. They were still there in the 1930s.[53] The only, though frequently economically and culturally problematic, alternative was to move to an over-expensive and socially unwelcoming municipal housing estate.[54]

The rush towards suburbia was not, of course, uniform or uniformly rapid. Larger numbers of people in smaller and poorer towns – the communities comprising the Black Country are a good example – which lacked a variegated social and occupational structure and a large and upwardly mobile professional class, remained clustered closer to the urban core than in large cities.[55] But every centre of any size boasted its own, distinctive suburban space.[56] The process of differentiation accelerated during the interwar period and even more so in the years after 1945.

How, then, did the emergence of a large-scale national suburbia fail significantly to modify the emphases and tonalities of the town–country dichotomy which has been described and interpreted in this chapter? First, a venerable urban–rural duality was reinforced by political developments in the early and mid-nineteenth century. Thus in terms of rhetoric, the debate over factory legislation, the crisis surrounding the great Reform Act of 1832 and extended inter- and intra-party conflict over free trade and the Corn Laws in the 1830s and 1840s, were invariably though superficially presented as epochal battles between the landed and the manufacturing classes. This greatly reinforced a cultural tendency to think and generalize within the context of exclusively rural or urban spheres. Second, and as a matter of fact rather than perception or political ideology, the growth of new towns between the 1780s and the 1840s – localities classically named 'shock cities' by Asa Briggs – had indeed been unprecedentedly rapid and disorienting.[57] As a consequence, paternalistic conservatives focused almost exclusively on the midlands and north, rather than pockets of abject poverty in much longer established centres or, crucially, on *spatial and occupational differences* between the shock cities themselves. This, also, tended subtly to exclude the suburban variable.

Third, the new industrial cities, which began to move towards a degree of political and administrative maturity in the mid-1830s, felt impelled stridently to assert their emergent identities over and against those of the landed elite – the so-called 'feudal' interest. The new and dynamic ideology of municipal government, predominantly articulated by civic leaders preoccupied by the task of reforming specifically inner city infrastructures, proved central to this discourse. As a consequence, the 'middle' – the by now rapidly expanding suburban sector – was once again tacitly excluded. Fourth, late nineteenth century and Edwardian metropolitan intellectuals invariably depicted the suburbs as irremediably philistine.[58] This critique combined with incessant attacks on the visual drabness of the new and rapidly expanding sector. The 'typical' suburb was said to lack a centre or 'heart', display an alienating architectural uniformity, and communicate neither the peace and quiet of the village nor – a paradox, this, given the ubiquity of pro-agrarian ideology – the exhilarating bustle of a crowded metropolitan or urban-industrial street.[59]

Finally, and astonishingly, only a minority of nineteenth century commentators drew attention to the fact that, from the very outset, some though by no means all suburbs adopted and mimicked the values and lifestyles *of* the countryside.[60] Later, of course, it would become a truism that preference for terrace or semi-detached rather than flat or apartment, dedication to garden or allotment, and, as time went on, commitment to bowls, cricket, tennis and Sunday park football, demonstrated enthusiasm not for a rural idyll but for a very particular kind of attachment to the country in the city. In reality, then, late nineteenth and earlier twentieth century suburbs constituted a bridge between the at least partly imagined polarity of country and city. But the imbedded resilience of a social and cultural discourse reaching back to the late medieval period, and rooted in intense distaste for the immorality, luxury and moral pollution of the capital, militated against a radical modification of the town–country dyad, a dichotomy which, as we have seen, profoundly shaped late nineteenth and twentieth century rural preservationism. This may seem an unremarkable conclusion. But only when the suburban variable has been more convincingly theorized and historicized within this context will it be possible to move towards an adequate account of an abiding cultural duality in modern and contemporary England and Britain.[61]

CHAPTER 9

ENVIRONMENTAL JUSTICE, HISTORY AND THE CITY: THE UNITED STATES AND BRITAIN, 1970-2000

Historians as activists?

This chapter explores linked issues in the historical sociology of academic knowledge. It seeks to unravel relationships between environmental activism and the shaping of national variants of environmental history.[1] Engaging with differences between recent developments in the United States and the United Kingdom, the chapter suggests that, in synchronization with the onset of a more overtly urban bias among grassroots activist movements, the environmental historical community in America evolved rapidly between the 1970s and the beginning of the new century. This thirty-year period witnessed animated interaction between overtly political concerns and divisive ideological and intellectual issues – particularly in relation to race, gender, cultural relativism and postmodernism.[2] The American sub-discipline expanded rapidly in term of numbers of practitioners and generated its own internal controversies, notably *vis-à-vis* the emergence of a distinctively urban-environmental as opposed to long-established agro-ecological lineage.[3] More recently, American historians have begun to engage with the concept of 'environmental justice', a term encapsulating commitment to the belief that insupportable discrepancies in quality of life experienced by inhabitants of deeply deprived inner city areas and an environmentally privileged suburbia must be radically narrowed.[4]

However, environmental justice means different things to different people. Adherents of what is here defined as the 'wide spectrum' approach, exemplified in this chapter by the work of Dolores Greenberg, believe that the concept should be brought into play to strengthen and legitimate contemporary political struggle. Scholars like Greenberg are also deeply committed to eradicating 'eco-racism', a concept based on the argument that to a far greater degree than any other socio-economically disadvantaged group it is people of colour, both historically and in the present, who have been most cynically subjected to life-threatening levels of urban degradation.[5] Here, as in other contexts, the 'class–race' dichotomy remains powerfully present in American historical and social scientific discourse. On the other hand, historians like Harold Platt, whose work is discussed in detail here, deploy environmental justice in a style which clearly differentiates between past and present and largely eschews direct reference to eco-racism. Platt argues that late nineteenth century urban reformers drew on quite different ideological, linguistic and cultural resources to those used by early twenty first century activists engaged in the battle for local, regional and national environmental equality.[6]

Environmental history in Britain during this period remained under-developed. Numbers of practitioners were small and distanced themselves from controversial theoretical and methodological debate. At the level of political activism, British, like American, environmental movements, appeared to become increasingly involved with urban issues. But in this chapter it is argued that change of this kind was more apparent than real. At the same time a deeply imbedded anti-urban-industrial ethos continued to be reflected in the preoccupations of the environmental historical community. Thus only in the 1990s would the sub-discipline generate overviews and monographs which began to do even cursory justice to key issues during the peak period of industrialization between the mid-nineteenth and early twentieth centuries.[7] We shall also note that, during the same decade, a minority within a minority of networks concerned with environmental activism, influenced by developments in the United States, began to undertake investigations into aspects of contemporary urban environmental justice.

Might we, then, be justified in assuming that environmental activists and historians in the United Kingdom will in the future devote increased attention to the urban variable? Not necessarily: fundamental historical and cultural differences, rooted in the differing intensity of ethnic conflict in the two countries during the last century and a half, will probably tend to make it less likely that eco-racism will be as ardently championed in Britain as in America. As a corollary, its natural bedmate – environmental injustice – will be likely to occupy a less prominent position in public and scholarly debate. However, this conclusion is not set in stone. For were British environmental historians finally to engage more enthusiastically with theoretical and methodological debate in the disciplinary mainstream, a much wider range of hitherto marginalized research topics, which do indeed relate to the issues of social, economic, and environmental equity in the nineteenth and twentieth century city, might establish themselves. In that sense, both for activists and historians, the future remains open. Much, however, will depend on the role played by the urban historical community in Britain, and the manner in which that long-established sub-discipline reacts to environmentally focused work that has been produced since the early 1990s. If British environmental scholars have too often remained blind to the urban variable, historians of the city have thus far resisted full engagement with methodologies and findings generated by the more youthful sub-discipline.

The process whereby the concept of environmental justice came to be partially appropriated by a small number of historians working on the late nineteenth and early twentieth American city is now well documented.[8] From the later 1970s urban activists grew increasingly impatient with traditional organizations such as the Sierra Club, National Wildlife Federation and National Audubon Society. These bodies were accused of being more concerned with threatened species and the preservation of wilderness than improvement in the conditions endured by city-dwellers forced to live in heavily degraded downtown neighbourhoods. Militants campaigned against toxicity-producing waste disposal policies, lead poisoning attributable to inner city highway construction and countless forms of industrial pollution. Gaining extensive media coverage in the aftermath of the much-publicized Love Canal, New York State and Warren County, North Carolina episodes in 1978 and 1982, direct action groups established local and then regional and national organizations.[9] Angry community reaction to corporate and governmental indifference to health threats in poor neighbourhoods contributed to an enhanced sense of empowerment. In time, environmental coalesced with broader political and feminist concerns.

Here, eco-racism constituted a powerful rallying-cry. As John Agyeman has noted, environmental issues between the 1970s and the beginning of the new century were redefined in terms of 'justice, equity and rights'. At the same time, the term 'environment' itself underwent discursive transformation, becoming a live issue for those who saw themselves as direct successors to the civil rights movement.[10] By the late 1980s, long-established pressure groups had started to incorporate radical grassroots strands into traditional agendas. Initially, it was argued that health-destroying pollution endured in poor communities, in which ethnic minorities were frequently over-represented, should be redistributed outwards towards the suburbs. However, a minority of activists now argued that the well-tried slogan 'not in my backyard' should be replaced by 'not in anyone's backyard'. Ecological and global discourses in this sense came to be more widely articulated. As Andrew Dobson has noted, a minority of activists began to adopt increasingly holistic political attitudes towards relationships between men, women and urban nature. Nevertheless, for a majority, the idea of environmental justice remained inextricably linked to the anti-eco-racist belief that white suburbanites enjoyed an unjustifiably and, so it was argued, 'unconstitutionally' superior quality of life to that endured by people of colour living in grossly degraded inner cities and run-down suburbs.[11] Conflicts of the latter type remained local and regional rather than ecological and global. In addition, it was argued by academics committed to environmental justice and opposition to eco-racism that increased local awareness of triggers of pollution crises served to empower the politically powerless. In turn, local conflict revealed the extent to which city, state and federal governments had manipulated political systems to conserve an inegalitarian status quo.

Urban-environmental history in the United States

Meanwhile, American environmental history went through several cycles of change. Traditionally defined in agro-ecological terms, in the early 1970s the sub-discipline began to engage with the city. Inspired by the pioneering research of Joel Tarr, and subsequently Martin Melosi and William Cronon, scholars investigated urban infrastructural and ecological issues.[12] From the 1980s onwards work informed by feminist principles complemented an increasing range of publications on public water supply, and sewage and garbage disposal systems. Drawing on historiographical developments rooted in the 1970s, researchers pointed to a distinctive women's role in relation to pollution, 'municipal housekeeping' and social reform.[13]

In addition, in the 1980s influential urban-environmental historians engaged with issues associated with post-modernism and cultural relativism. Thus far scholars had tended to assume that mountains, prairies, plains, streets, factories, sewers and rivers were indisputably 'out there', non-problematic phenomena unambiguously available to social-scientific investigation. However, developments in cultural, critical and literary theory, and in historical geography, now implied that such confidence could not be justified. Just as travel writers return from distant lands with divergent accounts of topography, agriculture, industry, and social structure, so environmental historians might need to acknowledge that different individuals or interest groups view the 'same' landscape or city in different ways. This debate about perspective, evidence and interpretation ended in compromise. Protagonists admitted the existence of a wide diversity of perceptual and ideological stances but refused to follow a relativist route that would have implied that accounts of environmental change can *only* be culturally determined. Rather than commit themselves to this agenda, a majority of scholars in the United States opted for the idea that a wide range of different narratives should be subjected to controlled interrogation.[14] The extent to which the environmental historical community in the United States was transformed by engagement in these intense theoretical and methodological interchanges should not be over-estimated. Just as many mainstream political historians in Britain ignored debates about postmodernism, cultural relativism and the linguistic and cultural turns, so many American environmental scholars ignored the 'theory wars'. At the same time, research into predominantly agro-ecological problems continued to prosper.

By the end of the twentieth century, environmental historians in the United States were producing very large numbers of case-studies of scientific, technological and systemic change; analyses of communal and legal conflict over pollution of air and water; and journals and monographs on economic and cultural tension between town and country. Much of this work was set within a broadly ecological and systems framework. Indeed, a case can be made for arguing that over-emphasis on the ecological variable may have played a role in persuading a small number of historians to turn, during that most recent cycle of debate, to the application of concepts derived from the environmental justice movement to the late nineteenth and early twentieth century American city.[15]

The image of the city as system appeared to have excluded an issue that had long preoccupied urban historians in the United States – the establishment, maintenance and deployment of political power which exerted a massive impact, either directly or indirectly, on collective quality of life and relative equity in terms of the distribution of economic, social, environmental and cultural resources. Appropriation of the concept of environmental injustice, it was argued, would allow direct engagement with the issue of equality – and, more specifically, who had benefited, and failed to benefit, from improvement in the provisions of urban housing and public utilities. It might also make it possible to gain a clearer understanding of how landlords, policy-makers and power-brokers had so effectively spatially segregated and regulated the urban sphere. Given the interactive nature of relationships between present and past, we should hardly be surprised that an approach claiming to show how injustice had been legitimated and reaffirmed in the contemporary American city began to exert a magnet-like attraction over members of the urban environmental community.

Thus in a persuasive contribution, Harold Platt draws on and modifies ideas derived from the environmental justice movement to reinterpret resistance on the part of corrupt city bosses and landlords to take action against sub-standard and disease-ridden working class housing. Platt points to the central role played by 'public policy ... in the degrading of the quality of life' and in spatially 'creating places [that were] below accepted standards of human health and decency'.[16] He claims to bring 'an environmental perspective to bear on urban politics that can help situate ethnicity, patronage, and [political] machines within broader, more inclusive, frameworks of analysis'.[17]

Platt interrogates the intolerable conditions endured by working-class inhabitants.

The key historical moment in Chicago proved to be a series of reformist investigations into a typhoid epidemic that ravaged the Nineteenth Ward in 1903 and which demonstrated that poverty-stricken areas were massively more likely than affluent suburbs to be afflicted by filth diseases. Platt argues that the strategy developed by the urban reformer Jane Addams, of 'exposing corruption by focusing public attention on carefully selected landlords and inspectors, was a logical and effective way to launch the struggle for environmental justice'.[18] However, Platt acknowledges the resilience of a deeply imbedded and corrupt party machine and admits that 'politicians simply moved their base of operations from the health to the building department which became the new den of thieves for loyal patronage workers'.[19]

Dolores Greenberg's survey of the reconstruction of race and protest in New York City is informed by what is termed in this chapter a 'wide spectrum' variant of the paradigm, a perspective which uses the historical chronicle of gross urban inequity explicitly to support the struggle for environmental justice in the here-and-now. Greenberg asserts that people of colour 'historically lacked protection of their most fundamental right – the right to life'.[20] Moreover, the legacy of slavery involved an 'inequitable distribution of well-being as old as the ecological transformation occasioned by the city's founding'.[21] Explicitly linking past to present, Greenberg insists that 'resistance movements founded on premises of social ecology articulated ... a reform agenda that bears remarkable similarities to current advocacy'.[22] During the earlier twentieth century New York witnessed 'environmental justice efforts driven by local attachments, organized by activists from inner-city neighbourhoods, supported by informal national networks, and motivated by the common purpose to redress enmeshed social, political, economic and ecological degradation'.[23] Militants are said to have created a 'heritage of national protest for by-passing racist political processes that sustained poverty, powerlessness and unequal protection'.[24]

Characterizing Harlem as an 'endangered habitat', Greenberg contends that, by the 1960s, the lessons of the past had persuaded environmental activists to participate in 'a historic first', not only in the contested district itself but 'around the world', with 'popular ecological resistance movements ... challeng[ing] fused inequities of place, governance, and distributive justice'. Greenberg goes on to argue that 'the wider culture's integration of the reform configuration became a force for social change that encouraged politically marginalized minorities to further strengthen protests against government failure to act on their own behalf'.[25] As in our own times, so in nineteenth and earlier twentieth century New York, 'everyday knowledge of inherited patterns of racism and spatial segregation shaped an awareness among people of colour of the connections between environmental and social systems governing their survival.'[26] Where Platt acknowledges the limits of the historical application of ideas derived from the environmental justice movement, Greenberg draws on urban, social and political history to bolster the struggle for urban equality in the early twenty first century. One variant of the environmental justice paradigm, represented by the Platt contribution, emphasizes the extent to which non-linearity complicates attempts to make one-to-one comparisons between the struggle for better conditions in the city in the late nineteenth and early twenty first centuries. The other, exemplified by Greenberg's article, seeks to persuade readers that the words, concepts and categories which energized radical action 150 years ago were astonishingly similar, indeed, sometimes *directly* 'led to', the making of the environmental justice movement in the here-and-now.

Greenberg's criticisms of Andrew Hurley's classic study of Gary, Indiana, bring these issues into full perspective.[27] Hurley's analysis demonstrates that fine-grained empirical research can frequently transform key activist landmarks into temporary way-stations. In Gary, repeated redrawing of the residential map interacted with the machiavellianism of managers at US Steel to ensure that ever-shifting sectors of the population became subjected to severe levels of atmospheric pollution. Environmental reform groups were established, fragmented, and then came together again. There was little linearity: as always, the past proved itself a different and unknown country. Hurley's portrait complicates the idea of triumphalist environmental victory, gives as much attention to progressive failure as to success and highlights the extent to which scientific expertise slowly but indisputably redefined communal perception of the epidemiological impact of a massive urban pollution problem.

As the inhabitants of the town gradually became aware of the extent of the damage inflicted on the community, increasingly sophisticated surveys of the long-term effects of uncontrolled pollution redefined the nature of the risk. At the very end of Hurley's period, US Steel found itself under increasing pressure both to make recompense for the misdemeanors of the past and to conform to enhanced technical-cum-environmental standards in the future. But, even in the 1990s, victory proved elusive: every step forward redefined the nature as well as the shape and thrust of protest. Hurley's study suggests that wide spectrum variants of the environmental justice paradigm oversimplify complex historical narratives.

In addition to underplaying the extent to which pollution problems are repeatedly redefined in the light of new scientific knowledge, the model works against a full understanding of shifting relationships between economic and occupational structure and the dynamics of opposition to corporate and governmental malpractice. Hurley's research also underlines the fact that linearity, progressivism, and idealization of the roles of individuals may well inhibit a fully contextualized understanding of environmental conflict.[28] In short, the wide spectrum paradigm favoured by Greenberg is better suited to the task of legitimating community empowerment in the present than explaining pollution problems in the past. This is not to denigrate social and political movements which seek to reduce appallingly inequitable levels of environmental degradation. Nor does a critique of this kind deny the widespread existence and influence of eco-racism. Rather, the aim is to ask questions about the nature and public function of history and its role in informing and underpinning the efforts of those engaged in environmental activism and to ask whether interpretative complexity must invariably and inevitably yield to the demands of progressive ideological unity.

Environmental history in Britain since 1970

As in the United States, environmental activism in Britain in the 1960s had long been dominated by conservative organizations such as the Council for the Preservation (later Protection) of Rural England, the National Trust and the World Wildlife Fund. These bodies had been heavily influenced by elitist preoccupations with the freezing of a purportedly 'untouched' nature.[29] Despite the activities of the Campaign for Nuclear Disarmament, protest against weapons of mass destruction was less developed and less effectively sustained than in other parts of Europe.[30] The founding of Greenpeace and Friends of the Earth in 1970–1 and 1977 generated higher levels of direct action. The former body coordinated demonstrations against a wide range of issues such as corporate indifference towards recycling, the industrialization of the whaling industry, Britain's independent nuclear deterrent and the cruelty of the fur trade. Friends of the Earth protested against American nuclear tests in Alaska, seal culling in Newfoundland and governmental waste disposal policies.[31]

Opposition to the construction of ever-larger numbers of motorways also increased during this period. Nevertheless, and despite the fact that the first European Green Party was founded in Britain in 1973, it is difficult to detect a strong association between rising memberships of environmental organizations and radical political change. In Germany, by contrast, parliamentary and extra-parliamentary protest made a significant impact on nuclear energy, toxic waste and highway construction policies. However, during the 1980s, and particularly in the aftermath of the rampantly pro-car policy statement, *Roads for Prosperity* (1989), a new kind of militancy began to achieve a more prominent public profile. The Earth First! Coalition held its first annual conference in 1992 and rapidly staked a claim as an umbrella coordinator of radical community action against motorway and airport construction, quarrying, open-cast mining and experimentation with genetically modified crops. As in the United States, long-established organizations now modified agendas long dominated by the preservation of nature and the protection of endangered species.

In the early 1990s alternative, loosely knit groups such as the Women's Environmental Network, the Black Environment Network and the Environmental Justice Network came into being. At the very end of the century, Friend of the Earth's 'Pollution Justice Campaign' began belatedly to target specifically urban issues. Claiming that over 650 of the largest factories in the United Kingdom were to be found close to residential areas with an average household income of less than £15,000 (€21,500), the survey confirmed that only five such plants had been established in localities in which families earning over £30,000 (or approximately €43,000) predominated.

Over 90 per cent of manufacturing plants in the London region were situated in districts characterized by below average household income while in the north-east more than four-fifths of large-scale manufacturing units were to be found in areas in which a majority of households earned no more than £5,000 (or approximately €7,010) a year.[32] This was the context within which new radical groups emphasized that traditional conservationist bodies had represented the interests of '[the] well-off, [the] white [and] middle-class'.[33] Appealing to 'community groups, networks, national and local organizations, schools and committed individuals', the Environmental Justice Network echoed the conclusions of the Friends of the Earth factory report and told its 600 affiliates that the 'poorest communities suffer the worst environments'.[34] To urban and environmental historians, these findings are, of course, unsurprising, indeed very nearly trivial. But that may be to miss the point. The significance of the report was its insistence that issues of this kind, which had thus far been wholly ignored both by British environmental movements and environmental historians, must finally be confronted.

Despite minority interventions of this kind, early twenty first century British environmental movements have continued to be heavily influenced by predominantly rural values. Thus a recent quantitative breakdown of themes dominating protests between 1988 and 1997 reveals that broadly non-urban almost certainly outnumbered broadly urban targets. The most prominent in the sphere as a whole was transport, with demonstrations against new motorways accounting for the bulk of interventions. Spurred on by quality of life issues in towns threatened by the ubiquitous culture of the private car, demonstrations of this kind were nevertheless underwritten by an intense desire to defend traditional village life, and intimately related to arcadian, anti-materialist and New Age ideals.[35] The environmental status of the city remained peripheral. The culture of an 'untouched' countryside, closely related to the continued political and cultural influence of the British upper and upper-middle classes as well as to the fact that so many members of the first industrial nation sought solace in a rural and arcadian vision of England, continued to predominate. The heritage and tourist industries also played a powerful and culturally reinforcing role.

What of British environmental history? In sharp contrast to events in the United States, between the 1970s and 1990s the sub-discipline remained in a state of suspended animation, largely oblivious to theoretical and methodological controversy within the disciplinary mainstream. Neither the 'limits of growth' debate of the 1970s nor the worldwide emergence of ecological discourses precipitated the formation of a specifically historical academic community.[36] In the small numbers of places in which it was practised the sub-discipline tended to be undertaken by geographers, geologist, climatologists and environmental scientists.[37] However, scholars working on the early modern period – preeminently Keith Thomas – published pioneering and invaluable studies of pre-modern attitudes towards nature.[38] Institutionally marginalized by economic, social and urban history, research into the environmental tended to be inhibited by long-standing barriers between 'science' and 'non-science' and the widely held belief that work in the field could only be undertaken by scholars whose major expertise was technical and scientific rather than historical.[39]

There may be another kind of explanation for the relative backwardness of environmental history in Britain in the period before approximately 1990. In the late 1970s it had been persuasively argued that the long-running standard of living debate would only be settled when larger numbers of researchers engaged with the issue of quality of life in the new industrial society.[40] Only a handful of historians took up the challenge and as a result broadly environmentally-orientated studies of individual towns remained thin on the ground.[41]

However, in due course, demographic historians and historical epidemiologists began to investigate the extent to which inequalities may have been directly or indirectly linked to maldistribution of urban resources and utilities. Such work has, *inter alia*, identified overcrowding as a key variable in relation both to the transmission and increased virulence of microorganisms responsible for the dissemination of specific diseases. Indeed, British scholars are now moving towards a point at which cause of death data can be used to illuminate historically elusive environmental variables. At the same time, environmental evidence is being deployed to throw light on the spatial incidence of bacteriologically and virally distinctive infections.[42] In addition, numerous studies of infant mortality have explored the roles played by class, occupation and locality in determining death rates among the youngest members of the community. Fine-grained analysis of individual household level data has made it possible to identify interactions between housing, incidence of breast-feeding and disposal of domestic waste.[43] It might therefore be hypothesized that the cultural space occupied by environmental history in the United States has been partially appropriated in Britain by demographic and epidemiological history.

Anglo-American contrasts

Only an arch-British patriot would deny that over the last 30 years environmental history has been dominated by American initiative and American innovation. Breaking with the preoccupation with wilderness studies, a pioneering group of scholars during the 1970s began to investigate urban networks and infrastructure. Engaging somewhat later with theoretical and methodological debate within the disciplinary mainstream, the new community revealed itself to be open to issues of gender. More recently, a small number of historians have begun to explore the potential of the environmental justice paradigm.

In Britain, on the other hand, the environmental historical community failed to expand, a state of affairs that may have been related to the dominant values underlying environmental activism, the failure, for whatever reason, of interested academics to make crucial connections between present and past, the pre-existing supremacy of economic, social and urban history and the institutionalized explosion of demographic, medical and epidemiological research.[44] During this period dominant strategies among environmental organizations ranged from the non-confrontational, through public demonstrations to one or another form of direct action.[45] However, the most influential, though invariably occluded, *leitmotif* continued to be either openly or tacitly rural. Even the intensification of radical protest during the 1990s has been more heavily influenced by preoccupation with the preservation of village culture than the now fully publicized plight of economically and socially excluded minorities in otherwise unprecedentedly affluent towns and cities.

In the United States political activism will undoubtedly ensure that the wide spectrum environmental justice paradigm becomes increasingly influential. Continuing to live out the contemporary repercussions of a deeply troubled racial past, and possessing a legal system which encourages citizens to seek equity through the courts in every sphere of communal life, America habitually looks, in its unending quest for the 'good' society, to a quite different set of mediating institutions than has evolved in Britain. In this sense, the environmental justice movement, and eco-racism, could only have attained political and cultural prominence in a nation, which has experienced and continues to live with the multiple legacies of the civil rights movement.[46] Will these traditions and linked ideological concerns enable protagonists of the wide spectrum paradigm to formulate convincing diagnoses of the inequalities of the urban past? Or will the inherently present-centred nature of this powerful ideology, exemplified by Greenberg's recent chapter, obscure the inherently non-linear historical processes that it seeks to clarify? The question remains open. But in Britain it is to be hoped that environmental historians will finally engage with sociological, ideological and methodological controversy, move closer to the disciplinary mainstream, and focus as intensively on the city – and inequality in the city – as on the countryside.

CHAPTER 10

PLACE, DISEASE AND QUALITY OF LIFE IN URBAN BRITAIN, 1800–1950

Cities in crisis, 1800–60

Among British cities in 1800 only London and Dublin had populations of more than 100,000: London a staggering round million, and Dublin 165,000. For the last 30 years 'new industrial districts' had expanded at an explosive rate but none had yet joined the 100,000 league: in 1800 there were 90,000 inhabitants in Manchester, 10,000 fewer in Liverpool.[1] Fifty years on, five more British towns had joined the demographic giants, with 15 others recording populations of more than 50,000.[2] In 1851, of the 12 largest urban centres in the 'known' world – excluding China? – no fewer than six (London, Liverpool, Manchester, Glasgow, Birmingham and Dublin) were to be found in England, Scotland or Ireland.[3]

Nearly six million Britons now called themselves town-dwellers. Non-industrial or commercial centres, crucial to economic and social change in the seventeenth and eighteenth centuries, had expanded less rapidly.[4] The population of freakish Bradford increased by 700 per cent between 1800 and 1850. At the other end of the scale, Exeter, Norwich, Chester and Shrewsbury failed to double in size. Shrewsbury grew by 30 per cent. Anomalously, 'partially industrialized' Nottingham failed to double its population during this same 50-year period.[5] By the turn of the twentieth century no fewer than 46 centres had joined the 100,000 club.[6] Newly promoted towns in the west Midlands included Walsall: in Yorkshire, Hull and Halifax: in Lancashire, Burnley and Preston and in Wales, Swansea. (A few years later, Merthyr Tydfil joined the biggest pace-setters.)[7] The speed of urbanization – and urban-industrialization – had been astonishing. In 1851 one out of every two inhabitants in England and Wales was recorded as resident in an urban location. Fifty years later, the figure had risen to seven out of ten and by 1950 four out of five.[8] In terms of large-scale urbanization, early twentieth century Germany trailed Britain by about 60 years. France lagged much further behind.[9]

As Tony Wrigley showed in a classic article more than half a century ago, London had long occupied a tier of its own. Wrigley concluded that the capital had a profound national demographic and epidemiological impact, dictated patterns of fashion, consumption and cultural change, and generated a mass market that played a crucial role in the transition from what Adam Smith called a commercial to a manufacturing society.[10] London has frequently occupied centre-stage in this book, and with good reason. The drama of the new industrial areas, and the way in which, in Asa Briggs's classic phrase, their 'shock' impact fascinated and appalled contemporaries, has been intensively discussed since the early nineteenth century.[11] For reasons of scale, the capital has proven analytically unmanageable. Its 'archaic' governing system, discussed in Chapter 5, has stretched the patience of even the most dedicated scholar seeking to understand relationships between economic, urban and epidemiological developments and the distribution of social and political power. Since the early nineteenth century millions of people have called themselves 'Londoners'. But the capital itself has remained something of a geographical and, viewed as a spatial totality, rather than a national seat of government or heart of the Empire, a cultural abstraction.[12] For the nineteenth and early twentieth centuries our greatest novelists – Dickens, Trollope, Gissing, James – are the best guides. For the Edwardian and interwar years there is no better fictional representation than Virginia Woolf's magnificent *The Years*.

The largest city in Europe, London numbered over 600,000 in 1700: a century later, a million. The population doubled again by 1850. In 1900 over six and half million people called themselves Londoners, and lived in the largest 'greater' administrative metropolitan region the world had ever seen.[13] In the second half of the nineteenth century the incorporation of towns and villages accelerated. Simultaneously, the capital went through a suburban revolution. In 1881 the southern district of Lambeth was home to more than a quarter of a million, neighbouring Wandsworth 210,000 and Camberwell 185,000. In 1851 Hackney, a highly desirable residential location for well-to-do eighteenth century merchants, housed 60,000 inhabitants, a figure that rose to more than a quarter of a million half a century later.[14] By the 1870s, the capital had engulfed large parts of the Hertfordshire, Kentish and Surrey countryside. Countless communities found themselves drawn into the octopus-like grip of the metropolis.

Within comfortable riding distance of the City to the south, in 1800 Croydon – a town that provides a running sub-theme in this chapter – clung to its ancient status as an independent market town. In 1830 only about 12,000 people lived there, a figure that rose to approximately 30,000 by 1860. At the beginning of the twentieth century Croydon's social elite continued to look upon the town (or suburb?) as an emphatically non-metropolitan community. However, by 1900, its population, like that of Hackney, had spiralled to a quarter of a million. One of the largest commuter areas in the world, Croydon had been colonized by builders and railway companies.[15] Seventy years earlier, a grumpy William Cobbett had ridden the road between London and the town and written of 'as ugly a bit of country as any in England. A poor spewy gravel with some clay. Few trees but elms, and those generally stripped up and villainously ugly.'[16] By 1900 stony road and elms had been replaced by segregated working- and middle-class streets and avenues, railway tracks, sidings and repair shops, and the occasional public park.

A century earlier many of those who commented on conditions in large towns were convinced that environmental problems in industrial Britain might become insoluble.[17] Anciently established urban elites were incapable of dealing with chronic infrastructural inadequacies. House-building lagged far behind an exponential increase in the demand for dwellings. Desperately high levels of over-crowding generated rampant levels of viral infection, particularly among the young. Failure to shift human waste from courts and alleys provided an ideal niche for deadly bacteria. These problems have been described in detail in Part 1.

Anthropometric historian Roderick Floud and his co-authors have concluded that the 'impact of urban growth ... led to decreases in average height as larger proportions of the working-class community were subjected to town life', the result of nutritional, environmental, economic and psychological stress.[18] In 1841 life expectation at birth in Manchester and Liverpool still hovered in the upper twenties, implying that health levels were as bad as they had been during some of the worst crises of the medieval period. Even at mid-century, large industrial centres in the north recorded figures well below the national average: 'little evidence [can be detected] of a significant improvement until the 1870s or 1880s on the situation prevailing in the 1850s'.[19] Recent scholarship has validated the central planks of the case mounted against early urban-industrialism (and Sir John Clapham) by the determinedly non-quantitative John and Barbara Hammond in the 1920s.[20]

As described in Chapter 4, cholera, the 'new plague', dominated political, social and medical thought and consciousness. The disease has continued to claim the attention of urban and epidemiological historians. Yet we still lack a comprehensive overview of the disease in nineteenth century Britain – only the first outbreak has received detailed treatment.[21] Relatively little has been written about the exceptionally dangerous epidemics of 1848–9 and 1853–4.[22] Urban and epidemiological historians have undertaken only limited city-specific research into the relationships between the pandemic infection and social and political instability.[23]

The 'Asiatic plague' claimed remarkably few victims compared with the leading killing infections of the early and mid-nineteenth century. As Margaret Pelling has shown, fever – confused with or thought to bear a strong familial relationship to cholera – claimed exceptionally large numbers of urban lives.[24] We have seen in Chapter 3 that by 'fever' medical men usually meant typhus or typhoid. The former struck whenever desperately deprived living standards declined yet further and, interacting with filthy domestic conditions, played into the hands of the human body louse. Typhus wrought havoc on a regional or national level and continued to linger – creating endemic niches – in over-crowded and semi-starving 'fever-haunts', when a large-scale outbreak had receded.[25] As for typhoid, it claimed exceptionally large numbers of lives between late summer and late autumn.

But neither condition was as destructive as tuberculosis, the biggest killer of adults throughout the nineteenth and earlier twentieth centuries.[26] However, it was deaths attributable to the 'inevitable' conditions of infancy and childhood which claimed the largest numbers of lives during our period. Measles, diphtheria, scarlet fever, whooping-cough and diarrhoea have been discussed in passing in several chapters in Part 1. Each was believed to have been partially domesticated in the eighteenth century. But intermittently, one or the other broke its endemic bounds and killed with ferocious intensity among the youngest and, in terms of resistance, least protected members of the community. Obsessed by adult mortality and the 'filth' diseases, early sanitarians gave little attention to 'everyday' infections. Led and dominated by Edwin Chadwick, they concentrated on the construction of what urban-environmental historians later came to call systems dedicated to the effective disposal of sewage and the provision of a reliable supply of unpolluted drinking water: the classic preventive barrier, sanitarians believed, against rampant and socially destabilizing outbreaks of cholera and typhus.

However, as we have seen in Chapter 6, the vision was flawed. Firstly, Chadwick's narrow-bored pipes created many more difficulties than they solved. Second, the agricultural disposal of sewage turned out to be a much more complicated business than utilitarian blue-prints suggested. Third, the circular system, combining water supply, sewage disposal and the use of human waste to boost agricultural production, required a far greater degree of coordination between town and country than the great majority of mid-nineteenth century communities were able or willing to muster. Finally, the weakness of Chadwick's epidemiological position – that outbreaks of disease could be monocausally explained in terms of interactions between emanations deriving from human and animal waste, and a generalized 'epidemic atmosphere' – failed to account for clear-cut differences in the observed pattern and behaviour of the wide range of conditions that triggered exceptionally high levels of mortality in early and mid-nineteenth century Britain.

Chadwick's reputation and national standing as sanitary supremo at the General Board of Health received a savage body blow at Croydon in the early 1850s. In 1852 the still putatively 'independent' community became known as a model sanitary town.[27] By the late summer of that year it had adopted a circular system, comprising water supply, tubular drainage, and the agricultural recycling of sewage. Almost immediately typhoid struck, and hit even harder in the early months of the following year – sometimes, in the right meteorological conditions, the 'autumn fever' continued to kill beyond its allotted span. There were 1,800 cases and 70 deaths in a population of 16,000. The outbreak coincided with the discovery of more than a hundred pipes blocked with 'flannel, hay, shavings, paper, hair, sticks, kittens, a night cap, a cat, pigs' entrails [and] a bullock's heart'.[28] Investigation followed investigation, several of them undertaken by engineers and sanitarians strongly committed to the Chadwickian cause. The pre-existing hygienic state of the town was blamed: so were lurking 'miasms', the general epidemic atmosphere, the state of the river Wandle, a neighbouring typhoid-prone village and the weather. Finally, a surprisingly plain-spoken survey concluded that Croydon's system had lacked adequate engineering expertise. Unnecessary economies had led to the laying of sub-standard, over-narrow pipes. There may even have been a strong spatial correlation between the incidence of typhoid and the location of the new sewers.[29] The evidence was damning.

After the waning of the Chadwickian star, Croydon persevered with its sanitary experimentation. The pace was set by Alfred Carpenter. Carpenter was a well-respected and influential medical man with a thriving practice in the town.[30] He never became medical officer of health but played a prominent and controversial role on the local board of health. A passionate advocate of the application of town waste to the land, in the early 1860s Carpenter emerged as the self-proclaimed 'director' of a large sewage farm at the nearby village of Beddington. From the 1860s onwards the population of Croydon soared – the market town had now indisputably been transformed into a massive outer metropolitan suburb. To preserve health, increasing volumes of sewage needed to be diluted by ever larger quantities of water. Controversy piled on controversy, with critics insisting that the well-being of the inhabitants of Croydon and Beddington had been compromised by fever: enteric and diarrhoeal infection attacked too hard and too frequently. In 1875 Croydon suffered another savage outbreak of typhoid, a haunting reminder of the tragedy of 1852–3. This time the death-toll reached into the nineties.[31] During the eighteenth century Croydon had been known for the purity of its 'waters' – the river Wandle 'teemed' with trout. No longer. Had seepage and leakage from Beddington worked their way into local watercourses? Were polluting workshops in the notorious Old Town to blame? Or had typhoid, dysentery and diarrhoea been repeatedly aerially transmitted into the community by the ubiquitous Beddington stench?

Carpenter stood firm. Neither a fully paid-up Chadwickian nor a proto-bacteriologist, he prepared statistical tables to show that, year in, year out, health levels in the two localities had improved. But nationally known scientists and sanitarians, and the townspeople of Croydon and the villagers of Beddington questioned the wisdom of the long-running sewage dilution experiment. Modifying theory and method to keep pace with changing ideas about the roles played by water, smell and seepage in the transmission of disease, Carpenter repeatedly came up with the same answer: dilution was good for health, good for farming, and good for Britain.[32]

His commitment to the large-scale application of sewage to agricultural land continued to be underwritten by an identical style of thinking to that championed by the numerous Chadwickian and post-Chadwickian reformers who have thronged the pages of Part 2 of this book. Carpenter favoured an economic, environmental and biological balance between town and country. But he remained a physiocrat – a nation's health depended on the well-being of its agriculture rather than industrial or commercial resilience. To critics who claimed that the 'sewage route' to the regeneration of the countryside had long been impracticable – large urban centres produced far too much human waste for the average farmer's financial capacities or the scale of his fertilizing needs – Carpenter responded that town councils might sometimes need to provide a small subsidy for the disposal of town sewage. Overheads were low and subsidies would be short-term, rarely involving a rate rise of more than a penny in the pound.

Benefits would be inestimable. Above all, the use of the dilution method would generate far-reaching qualitative change in the health and saleability of livestock raised on sewage-enriched fodder. The ever-enthusiastic Carpenter informed his readers that Beddington's unusually plump and healthy herds greedily gorged on rich Italian rye-grass: 'sleek and glossy', their flesh was as 'firm, and their contour and general appearance such as must delight the sight of the good farmer'.[33] Once again confronting the doubting inhabitants of Croydon, he pointed to the testimony of (unnamed) 'experts' who had confirmed that Beddington meat was 'exceedingly tender and juicy ... no epicure could wish for a better joint'.[34] What were minor amenity problems when measured against the possibility of the creation of an agrarian paradise?

A courageous optimism, 1860–1900

In the second half of the nineteenth century, intensive construction of infrastructure – particularly water and sewage treatment and disposal plant – significantly reduced the intensity of the environmental and epidemiological problems that had beset urban Britain between the 1780s and the 1860s. During this period '... urban improvers [were] active in building sanitary works, not as rapidly or as systematically as Chadwick would have liked, but on the whole successfully'.[35] The health dictator was sidelined for the rest of his life, a lone voice insisting that 'all disease is smell, all smell disease' and deaf to important advances in scientific, medical and technological knowledge and sanitary engineering. The generation following his fall from power – the 1850s to the 1880s – witnessed a strengthening of the idea, first propounded by John Snow and William Budd, that polluted water, rather than generalized effluvia, probably constituted the primary transmitter of cholera and typhoid.[36] The same period saw increasing numbers of scientists and medical men feeling their way towards a belief in the specificity of individual infective entities, rather than viewing the disease process as a sequence of interlinked and interchangeable gradations that changed according to the presence or absence of 'filth' and a vaguely defined (and intensively moralized) set of predisposing circumstances.

Debates about the relationship between water, dirt and hygiene continued, but in terms that gradually displaced the Chadwickian model. Edward Frankland, chemist, water analyst, and influential member of the Rivers Pollution Commission, agonized over the problem of 'previous sewage contamination': once 'touched' by human waste, Frankland believed, a specific source might never again be free from infection-bearing poison. Deep down, Frankland was convinced that 'doubtful' supplies should never be used. Nevertheless, he played a leading role in advocating the adoption of more rigorous selection techniques, safer storage systems, and controlled filtration procedures on the part of the metropolitan water companies.[37] Perhaps *some* contaminated sources could be repurified?

The cholera and fever years had taken a heavy toll. Pessimism – the fear that another catastrophic and 'plague-like' disease might devastate the greatest urban-industrial nation in the world – held sway until the early 1870s. But as emphasized in Chapter 1, among a minority, guarded optimism began to gain ground. Writing as early as 1859 about the final epidemic of bubonic plague in the capital in 1665 William Farr summoned up distressing images of 'loud voices, shrieks and sobs', 'raving patients', forced to rush out of their houses to escape the 'prison' of death in which they had found themselves incarcerated. Would London, and the new manufacturing centres, ever again experience such extremes of panic and horror? Farr thought not: urban civilization would survive. Improved diet, drainage, 'sound sanitary doctrines', and a more reliable water supply accounted for the many advances that had taken place since the first – plague-like – outbreak of cholera in 1831–2. Farr portrayed a roseate future in which '. . . a field of terror [would become] a field of health, concourse and security' to the 'population of the Metropolis of the Empire and Britain's other great towns and cities'.[38]

Six years later Farr found himself confronted by 'plague-like' conditions in the East End of London. He chronicled the experiences of cholera-stricken inhabitants in the worst hit areas, the brave efforts of a small number of public health officials and doctors to comfort the sick and dying, and babies and toddlers sinking into unconsciousness in their parents' arms. 'The sick were most patient', Farr reported, 'most willing to help each other, the women always in front, and never stinting danger. There is no desertion of children, husbands, wives, fathers, or mothers from fear.'[39] A year earlier, with the pandemic infection already threatening the continent, Farr had pondered the relationship between the monitoring of disease, social cohesiveness and civic order. Advocating 'open statistical government', he concluded that it was 'a common notion on the Continent that the publication of weekly tables, such as those of London, may shake the nerves of the people, and lead to terror in times of epidemic'.[40] In Farr's view, 'experience [proved] that the publication of the facts quiets instead of disturbing the popular mind, and while it reveals the exact extent of danger, robs it of the halo of alarm with which the imagination surrounds indefinite pestilences, walking abroad by noonday.'[41] A sense of optimism could only be nurtured if local and central government faced up to the facts of disease and confessed that, when an epidemic struck, the rising curve of mortality implied a near-criminal dereliction of duty. Potentially terrifying statistical information sternly underlined the necessity of repeatedly heightening sanitary vigilance.

Was Farr's sense of optimism in the midst of widespread death and suffering justified? Could towns and cities terrified and punished by cholera in 1831–2, 1848–9, 1853–4 and, now again in 1866 really be about to enter into a 'field of health, concourse and security'? There was evidence to the contrary, not least inability or unwillingness to care for the most vulnerable members of the community – the poor and poverty-stricken. During the cholera crisis of 1866 the medical officer for Bethnal Green recorded that his vestry had established an emergency committee that had entered into negotiations with selected medical assistants to ensure that surgeries would remain permanently open for the 'gratuitous supply of medicine'. 'The question of remuneration [was to be left] until the termination of their duties.'

Having considered the vestry's offer, the temporary appointees demanded £2 a day: the vestry refused to bargain and the plan collapsed. Next, the renting of a building to act as a temporary hospital foundered in the face of opposition on the part of local householders. Seventy sick paupers found themselves herded into the corridors of the workhouse infirmary. The guardians purchased an 'iron building' from the Fever Hospital and attempted to move healthy inmates out of the workhouse by offering single individuals three shillings a week and couples 4s 6d. Nevertheless, and despite the continuing epidemic, officials demanded that every new, uninfected applicant must formally 'enter the house' before being granted temporary outdoor relief. Rigid rules remained rigidly in place. Different parts of the metropolitan and local health systems went their different and random ways and failed to adjust to the needs of poverty-stricken members of the community trapped in an epidemic hell.[42]

Another example. In London between 1868 and 1870 twice as many individuals, most of them infants and children, died from scarlet fever as during the final epidemic of cholera. Conventional sanitary intervention failed to make an impact on the spread of the disease or the suffering that the prolonged outbreak brought to thousand upon thousand of working- and many middle-class families. The *Builder* admitted that little could be done about this 'alarming prevalence and spread of the fever'.[43] Long imbedded moralizing attitudes continued to set the tone. Working-class victims of the disease were accused of 'genuine and culpable carelessness', 'deliberate refusal to separate the healthy from the sick' and the 'grave moral offence' of neglecting to adopt 'practical means of preventing the spread of [every kind of contagious disease]'.[44]

Working people in exceptionally deprived areas of the capital were condemned for having done nothing to dissuade infected children from mingling with healthy friends on the landings of shared accommodation. There had even been attempts to prevent the removal of sick members of families to the Fever Hospital. Working-class inhabitants were blamed for 'resolutely [objecting] to the overpowering odour of the most effectual of the disinfectants, chlorine and carbolic acid' and 'loiter[ing] in the streets while their rooms were being fumigated, thereby 'carrying the disease elsewhere'.[45] The medical officer for Mile End concluded that in the future it would be necessary to introduce such 'stringent measures that it would be difficult to obtain authority for their acceptance'. The liberty of the individual – and particularly of the working-classes – would need to be circumscribed, lest 'mere tampering measures' encouraged the 'prolongation' of the next outbreak of disease.[46] Stressing legislatively-authenticated cooperation rather than coercion, John Simon chose his words more carefully. 'The public [might have to be] prepared to enforce thoroughly strict isolation rules.'[47]

While local elites and bureaucracies blamed the poor for their own suffering, progressive public health reformers continued to concentrate on the problem of prevention. Public utilities – particularly water supplies – must be more intensively monitored, the virtues of personal and collective hygiene reinforced, and larger numbers of infected individuals humanely isolated in fever hospitals. If measures of this kind could be made to bite, the diseases that had ravaged early and mid-Victorian Britain might be eradicated. As we have seen, some but by no means all these hopes were realized. The mid-1860s witnessed Britain's final large-scale outbreak of cholera. Typhoid survived into the twentieth century. But the 'water-route', capable of disseminating the disease over considerable distances, became less prominent: transmission via milk, shellfish, ice-cream and the immune carrier now came to the fore.[48] Dysentery declined and became less virulent than in the early and mid-nineteenth century when supplies of water had all too frequently been fetidly undrinkable.[49]

A majority of medical officers throughout the country now spoke of 'poisons', 'germs' and 'fungi', though others clung to modified versions of Chadwickian orthodoxy and attempted to fit new ideas about transmission into familiar sanitary frameworks.[50] By the 1880s it was becoming widely acknowledged that water played either a decisive, or powerful contextual, role in transmitting cholera, typhoid, dysentery and diarrhoea. Michael Worboys concludes that 'bacterial germ theories of disease became the *lingua franca* of public health medicine between 1880 and 1900'.[51] However, the mode of transmission of conditions like measles, diphtheria and scarlet fever remained mysterious. The same was true of bronchial and pneumonic infections, which struck with ferocity among the very young and the elderly. An impressive dossier of city-specific empirical information clarifying aspects of the causation and possible mode of spread of summer infant diarrhoea became more widely available. But death rates from the deadly seasonal condition – and differentials in levels of infant mortality in different urban centres – remained high.[52]

Micro-studies of poverty, pollution and housing, initially in London and then in other large centres, confirmed that each of the conditions which annually claimed so many adult, child and infant lives almost certainly possessed a specific and unique identity. Detailed analyses of serious outbreaks of disease, particularly those undertaken by the Local Government Board, generated an impressive store of information about the transmission of infection in a wide range of environments – urban, suburban and rural.[53] During the final 30 years of the century, William Farr's dream of the possibility of constructing a predictive science of epidemiology gave ground to an approach that deductively drew on data from numerous outbreaks of infection to identify the kinds of poisons, germs or bacteria that might be involved in specific localities. All this carried more weight than laboratory science or a largely imagined 'bacteriological revolution'.[54]

Every major centre made progress. However, there were significant differences between each of the demographic giants. In terms of life expectation at birth, London gained six years (38 to 44), Liverpool seven (31 to 38), Manchester four (32 to 36) and Birmingham five (37 to 42). Among northern industrial towns, Liverpool and Manchester recorded the smallest improvements between 1851 and 1900. The latter performed particularly badly: its 'mortality conditions in the 1890s were apparently little better in absolute terms' than they had been in Bradford, Leeds, Newcastle/Gateshead and Sheffield in the 1850s. This is brought into even sharper focus when it is noted that Manchester (and Liverpool) lagged a full decade behind the national average in the 1850s and 1860s. Nevertheless, by the end of the century, both cities had lifted themselves out of the abject conditions that had prevailed between 1820 and the 1860s. A corner had been turned.[55]

Twisting paths to progress: 1900–50

There was no linear path to healthier twentieth century urban living. As death rates fell, expectations rose and new problems emerged. Increasingly sophisticated methods of epidemiological analysis developed between the 1890s and the outbreak of World War I. Public health specialists focused on a wider range of variables and interactions – cause-specific morbidity, relationships between unemployment, poverty and illness: fine-grained differentials within and between specific districts: and comparisons of poverty-ridden locations with upper and middle-class norms. The health of infants and mothers came under increasingly intensive scrutiny.[56]

In many parts of the country, progress made between the 1880s and 1914 juddered to a halt at the end of World War I. In the 1920s and 1930s primary-producing sectors of the economy stuttered before plunging into depression. Social reformers in severely affected regions analysed epidemiological data and concluded that, compared with the capital and the south-east, industrial Britain had slipped back. Many areas – Glasgow, Newcastle, Belfast and socially deprived districts at the heart of the capital and in the East End – felt the full lash of poverty. Relativities came to the fore. Debates about the north–south divide entered a new phase, and sustained themselves in changing form up to and beyond the Black Report, published in 1988.[57]

A close reading of conditions in different urban typologies in the Barlow Report on the *Distribution of the Industrial Population*, published in 1940, reveals wide variations in interwar health. The committee concluded that wherever primary-producing industry had provided the nineteenth century economic and social ballast, unemployment, greatly reduced incomes, and reductions in aggregate local and regional demand, had wrought massive damage.[58] In J.B. Priestley's 'new England', dominated by light engineering, motor cars, charabancs, cheap mortgages and a novel range of electrical goods and consumer durables, indicators moved in the right direction.[59] Suburbia fared well, even in cities that had experienced the full shock of large-scale unemployment. The inhabitants of well-to-do houses lining the anonymous roads that now reached out from Manchester to the borders of the Cheshire countryside enjoyed good health. Even here, however, there were mixed areas. Just off the main streets of respectable and well-to-do Didsbury rack-rented and multi-occupied accommodation housed deprived sub-communities, with families of six sharing a single room.[60] In inner-city Hulme conditions were worse. High levels of unemployment and the survival of slum housing kept death and morbidity rates exceptionally high.[61]

In 1933 two neighbouring towns on Merseyside – Wigan and St Helens –recorded infant mortality rates of 110 and 116 per 1,000 live births. In the same year, the figures for Brighton and Oxford were 47 and 32.[62] At the very heart of affluent Britain, Kensington should have been healthier than Brighton and Oxford. Not so. The district had always been a socially and economically complex part of London.

To the south – in Brompton, Holland Park and Queen's Gate – could be found some of the finest homes in the land. To the north, unemployment, poverty, sub-standard housing, inflated rents and high levels of transience nurtured illness and premature death. At sub-district level in the south in 1932, Brompton and Queen's Gate recorded infant mortality rates of 11 and 12 per 1,000 live births – less than half the figure in Brighton: astonishingly, only two infants or toddlers were recorded as dying from infection in these areas in that calendar year. To the north, conditions were desperately bad. Both Golborne and Norland recorded infant mortality rates of more than 70 – double the Brighton figure. In Golborne infection accounted for more than half the deaths.[63]

Nor had interwar urban Britain yet been liberated from water and 'filth' transmitted outbreaks of disease. These could kill between 40 and a hundred people. In October 1937 Croydon experienced another severe outbreak of typhoid. The epidemic spread for another six weeks, finally accounting for 310 cases and 42 fatalities. Ancient memories were revived: in addition to the 'vast national scandal' of 1852–3, the town had, as we have seen, suffered a severe outbreak in 1875.[64] A community-backed South Croydon Typhoid Outbreak Committee demanded a public inquiry. The tribunal report rested on a style of epidemiological analysis that differed surprisingly little from a classic Local Government Board inquiry of the 1880s.[65]

Proposing and excluding a range of rival and-or potentially contradictory hypotheses, investigators concluded that a single workman – probably a carrier of the disease since World War I – had triggered the epidemic. The isolated labourer, suffering from a stomach upset, had no access to a toilet, and had been forced to use a bucket. The well, which fed into the town's supply, became tainted.[66] The tribunal's recommendations were addressed to a much wider range of agencies and individuals than would have been the case in the late nineteenth and earlier twentieth centuries. The borough engineer, council sub-committees and individual councillors, bacteriological laboratories, general practitioners, and water companies and their engineers and scientific advisors, were all taken to task.

The tribunal concluded that the medical officer had failed to keep in regular touch with the committee responsible for water supply. Nobody had told the borough engineer that chlorination had been suspended while building work was in progress. Local GPs were criticized for failing to contact the medical officer when patients first began to arrive at their surgeries complaining of stomach pains and diarrhoea. Finally, the building company was accused of irresponsibly failing to provide toilet facilities for the unfortunate workman. The committee recommended that a new set of official regulations be framed requiring the erection of temporary toilets during repair work in close proximity to reservoirs, wells and treatment works. A Widal test should be provided for any employee who had recently been suffering from a stomach problem.[67]

In 1945 the medical officer and senior public health officials in Croydon looked towards a brighter future. The spectre of diarrhoeal and enteric infection had finally been banished.[68] By the early 1950s, the infant mortality rate had stabilized in the lower twenties. In the mid- and late 1930s, it had been much higher, rising from 35 per 1,000 live births in 1935 to 60 in 1937 – the latter rate nearly twice as high as that recorded in the economically and environmentally privileged city of Oxford.[69] Prematurity replaced diarrhoeal and respiratory infections and 'other causes' as the leading category of early death among the youngest members of the community.[70] Nevertheless, as in the 1920s and 1930s, so in the late 1940s, intra-urban differentials remained worryingly high. Families in the inner areas of Central, Broad Green and Upper Norwood experienced infant mortality rates of 84, 95 and 75, only a fifth lower than those in St Helens and Wigan during the worst years of the 1930s.[71]

Following the stress and social dislocation of the war, tuberculosis remained a problem – in 1945 the medical officer noted that many poorer members of the community displayed a dangerous 'lowering of vitality', the result, he believed, of 'shortages of fats and milks'.[72] Five years later, nearly every form of the disease had been brought under much tighter control: the death rate from tuberculosis in 'great towns' (a venerable and unchanged Victorian category) sank to

0.42 per 1,000 population, in Croydon a mere 0.27.[73] Cancer and heart and circulatory diseases now accounted for more than 60 per cent of the town's annual death toll.[74] National urban mortality patterns had been transformed.

Croydon had long prided itself on its respectability. In the mid-twentieth century, the town's social elite continued to endorse a new suburban variant of that sacred ethos. However, like many other British towns, Croydon was a complex and mixed community. Following the establishment of the NHS, the health and epidemiological bars were raised. Prevention, now more frequently referred to as preventive medicine, still held the key to a better future. Above all, it was imperative to eradicate what had once been called 'fever haunts'. In 1954 a report on slum clearance – the first since 1931 – recorded that during the preceding 20 years separate dwellings in Croydon had increased by more than a quarter. However, very large numbers of multi-occupied houses lacked access to what the Labour government had designated the 'essential' amenities. Five thousand families or individuals in the town – or socially mixed suburb? – still shared a W.C., and 11,000 had no bath. Six thousand lacked access to a kitchen sink.[75] Little wonder that in 1952 the town's medical officer – speaking in tones similar to those of a late nineteenth century health reformer – reminded his readers that the 'fundamental importance of the work of the Sanitary Inspectors remains unchanged'.[76]

In the mid-1950s statutory health agencies joined forces with a staggeringly wide range of voluntary organizations – the Marriage Guidance Council, the Association of Moral Welfare, the Guild of Social Service and the Women's Voluntary Service – to tackle an age-old phenomenon: 'the problem family'. The medical officer praised the 'shining virtue' of deserted mothers who were claimed to have held house and home together. However, a large proportion of this caring core of the community were assumed to be of 'very mediocre intelligence'. No evidence was provided to support this conclusion, nor the assertion that nearly every father in families of this kind had renounced all responsibility for the well-being of his children. Perhaps, officials pondered, universal access to National Assistance benefit and Family Allowance had made a bad situation worse? One thing was certain. Mothers must not be evicted. It was as vital in the 1950s as in the 1870s that the health of 'the pivot of the family' be protected and improved.[77] Class- and morally-inflected attitudes and stereotypes endured. But they were expressed in less strident form than in the nineteenth and earlier twentieth centuries.

NOTES

Chapter 1   Country, Town and 'Planet' in Britain 1800–1950

1. However, there were already a small number of monographs concerned with historical aspects of environmental change, as well as studies dealing with the stewardship of nature. See in particular, on the early modern period, the classic Keith Thomas, *Religion and the Decline of Magic: Studies in Popular Beliefs in Sixteenth and Seventeenth Century England* (London: Weidenfeld and Nicolson, 1971), ch. 1 and on stewardship, John Passmore, *Man's Responsibility for Nature* (London: Duckworth, 1974). In 'The Alkali Act Administration 1863–84: the emergence of the civil scientist', *Victorian Studies*, 9 (1965), 85–112, Roy MacLeod entered unknown territory at a remarkably early date.

2. Important exceptions include Erwin Ackerknecht and George Rosen. See E.H. Ackerknecht, 'Anticontagionism between 1821 and 1876', *Bulletin of the History of Medicine*, 22 (1948), 562–93 and Ackerknecht, *History and Geography of the Most Important Diseases* (New York: Hafner, 1965). See, also, George Rosen, *A History of Public Health* (New York: MD Publications, 1958) and Rosen, 'Disease, debility and death' in H.J. Dyos and Michael Wolff (eds), *The Victorian City: Images and Reality: Volume Two* (London: Routledge and Kegan Paul, 1973), 625–67.

3. On the history of the patient, Roy Porter set the pace. See Roy Porter, 'The patient's view', *Theory and Society*, 14 (1985), 175–98 and Dorothy Porter and Roy Porter, *Patient's Progress: Doctors and Doctoring in Eighteenth Century England* (Oxford: Polity Press, 1989) For a survey of developments between the publication of the Porters' contributions and the near-present see Flurin Condrau, 'The patient meets the clinical gaze', *Social History of Medicine*, 20 (2007), 525–40.

4. The British Society for the Social History of Medicine led the way. Its *Bulletin* began publication in 1970, to be followed in 1988 by *Social History of Medicine*. The time was ripe for exploration of the 'social'. In the United States the *Journal of Social History* began publication remarkably early – in 1967. In the UK *Social History* followed, but not until 1976.

5. A provocative contributor has been Roger Cooter. See Roger Cooter, '"Framing" the end of the social history of medicine' in Frank Huisman and John Harley Warner (eds), *Locating Medical History: The Stories and their Meanings* (Baltimore: Johns Hopkins University Press, 2004), 309–37 and the same author's 'After death/after-"life": the social history of medicine in post-postmodernity', *Social History of Medicine*, 20 (2007), 441–64.

6. Michel Foucault's name began to climb the citation charts in the 1990s and has continued to do so. See Olga Amsterdamska and Anja Hiddinga, 'Trading zones or citadels? Professionalization and intellectual change in the history of medicine', in Huisman and Warner, *Locating Medical History*, 252.

7. However, Stephen Mosley has recently made the case for closer links between the social and the environmental. See Stephen Mosley, 'Common ground: integrating social and environmental history', *Journal of Social History*, 39 (2006), 915–33.

8. The key text is T.S. McKeown and R.G. Record, 'Reasons for the decline in mortality in England and Wales during the nineteenth century', *Population Studies*, 16 (1962), 94–122. This article has over a thousand citations and a thousand related items on Google Scholar. The McKeown paradigm has generated a vast literature. For succinct summaries and bibliographies see Bernard Harris, 'Public health, nutrition and the decline of mortality: the McKeown thesis revisited', *Social History of Medicine*, 17 (2004), 379–407 and Graham Mooney, 'Historical demography and epidemiology: the meta-narrative challenge', in Mark Jackson (ed.), *Oxford Handbook of the History of Medicine* (Oxford: Oxford University Press, 2011), 380–2.

9. Thomas McKeown, *The Modern Rise of Population* (London: Edward Arnold, 1976).

10. See, on this and related themes, Thomas McKeown, *The Role of Medicine. Dream Mirage or Nemesis?* (Oxford: Blackwell,1979) and his final book, *The Origins of Human Disease* (Oxford: Blackwell, 1988), which argues that in developing countries redistribution of wealth and income and improved methods of environmental intervention rather than 'modern medicine' point the way towards a less disease-ravaged future.

11. R.A. Lewis, *Edwin Chadwick and the Public Health Movement 1832–1854* (London: Longmans, Green, 1952): S.E. Finer, *The Life and Times of Sir Edwin Chadwick* (London: Methuen, 1952) and R.S. Lambert, *Sir John Simon 1816–1904 and English Social Administration* (London: MacGibbon and Kee, 1963).

12. Hobsbawm's evolving position can be traced in E.J. Hobsbawm, *Labouring Men: Studies in the History of Labour* (London:Weidenfeld and Nicolson,1968), chs 5–7. See, also, E.J. Hobsbawm, 'The British standard of living, 1790–1850' in A. J. Taylor (ed.), *The Standard of Living in Britain in the Industrial Revolution* (London: Methuen, 1975), 58–92.

13. The Hammonds' position is surveyed in Stewart A. Weaver, *The Hammonds: A Marriage in History* (Stanford: Stanford University Press, 1997): see, in particular, pp. 128–50. For the Hammonds' massive impact on twentieth

century social history see R.M. Hartwell, 'The rise of modern industry' in Hartwell, *The Industrial Revolution and Economic Growth* (London: Methuen, 1971), 377–89.

14. J.L. Hammond, 'The industrial revolution and discontent', *Economic History Review*, 1 (1930), 215–28. See, also, Weaver, *Hammonds*, 194–210.

15. A key moment was the United Nations Conference on the Human Environment in Stockholm in 1972. See *Development and Environment: Report of the United Nations Conference on the Human Environment* (The Hague: Mouton, 1972). By the end of the decade James Lovelock had published *Gaia: A New Look at Life on Earth* (Oxford: Oxford University Press, 1979). For 'globalism' in its many forms at this time see Niall Ferguson *et al., The Shock of the Global: The 1970s in Perspective* (Cambridge, Mass: Harvard University: The Belknap Press, 2010) and, particularly in the present context, J.R. McNeill, 'The environment, environmentalism and international society in the long 1970s', 263–78.

16. Guy Ortalano, *The Two Cultures Controversy: Science, Literature and Politics in Postwar Britain* (Cambridge: Cambridge University Press, 2009).

17. At the LSE I was advised to steer clear of the history of pollution and disease and concentrate on the (equally intriguing) topic of nineteenth century domestic service.

18. Joel Tarr's pioneering essays have been brought together in *The Search for the Ultimate Sink: Urban Pollution in Historical Perspective* (Akron, Ohio: University of Akron Press, 1996). In the 1980s and 1990s, his major themes were developed and extended by Martin Melosi. See Martin V. Melosi (ed.), *Pollution and Reform in American Cities 1870–1930* (Austin Texas: University of Texas Press, 1980); Melosi, *Garbage in the Cities: Refuse, Reform and the Environment* (College Station, Texas: Texas A&M University Press, 1981); and, a summation and extension of his earlier work, Martin V. Melosi, *The Sanitary City: Environmental Services in Urban America from Colonial Times to the Present* (Pittsburgh PA: University of Pittsburgh Press, 2000.) Mention must also be made of William Cronon's magisterial *Nature's Metropolis: Chicago and the Great West* (New York: Norton, 1991). By this point, American urban-environmental history had become a major academic growth-point.

19. For a very useful survey of European developments see Genevieve Massard-Guilbaud and Peter Thorsheim (eds), 'European Environmental History', *Journal of Urban History*, 33 (2007), 691–881. Special Issue. See, also, Dieter Schott, 'Resources of the city: towards a European urban environmental history' in Dieter Schott, Bill Luckin and Genevieve Massard-Guilbaud (eds), *Resources of the City: Contributions to an Environmental History of Modern Europe* (Aldershot: Ashgate, 2005), 1–27.

20. In his indispensable *The Demography of Victorian England and Wales* (Cambridge: Cambridge University Press, 2000), 340 and 352–3, the late Robert Woods made a case for exploring the proposition that the long-term decline of tuberculosis may also have been partly attributable to an autonomous change in virulence.

21. In 1974 Alan Armstrong made a move towards charting the spatial incidence of disease in his *Stability and Change in an English Town: A Social Study of York* (Cambridge: Cambridge University Press, 1974), 108–54. A decade later Robert Woods and John Woodward (eds), *Urban Disease and Mortality in Nineteenth Century England* (London: Batsford, 1984) included several contributions of a similar type. See in particular the chapters by Barbara Thompson on Bradford, Marilyn E. Pooley and Colin G. Pooley on Manchester and Robert Woods on Birmingham.

22. Typhoid deserves more intensive scrutiny. However, see Anne Hardy, *The Epidemic Streets: Infectious Disease and the Rise of Preventive Medicine* 1856–1900 (Oxford: Clarendon Press, 1993), 151–90 and an excellent recent thesis on the incidence of the disease, with reference to milk, and the development of different styles of epidemiological analysis. See Jacob Steere-Williams, 'The perfect food and the filth disease: milk, typhoid fever and the science of state medicine in Victorian Britain, 1850–1900', Ph.D. thesis, University of Minnesota, 2011. In addition, see Jacob Steere-Williams, 'The perfect food and the filth disease: milk-borne typhoid and epidemiological practice in late Victorian Britain', *Journal of the History of Medicine and Allied Sciences*, 65 (2010), 514–45.

23. This approach would be greatly refined in the mid-1990s by the 'Mortality in the Metropolis 1860–1920' project at the Centre of Metropolitan History, University of London. The project, funded by the Wellcome Trust, was undertaken with Graham Mooney and Andrea Tanner under the incisive administrative leadership of Derek Keene. Graham Mooney made several invaluable methodological breakthroughs during this five-year period. For an overview of some aspects of the work undertaken at that time see Graham Mooney, Bill Luckin and Andrea Tanner, 'Patient pathways: solving the problem of institutional mortality in London during the later nineteenth century', *Social History of Medicine*, 12 (1999), 227–70.

24. The best long period account of typhus in Britain remains Charles Creighton, *The History of Epidemics in Britain: Volume 2.* (London: Cass, 1965), 188–98. Edited by D.E.C. Eversley. See, also, Hardy, *Epidemics Streets*, 191–210 and J. D. Post, *The Last Great Subsistence Crisis in the Western World* (Baltimore: Johns Hopkins University Press, 1977), 129–32.

25. See E. Margaret Crawford, 'Typhus in nineteenth century Ireland' in Greta Jones and Elizabeth Malcolm (eds), *Medicine, Disease and the State in Ireland 1650–1940* (Cork: Cork University Press, 1999), 121–37.

26. Anne Hardy, '"Urban famine or urban crisis?": typhus in the Victorian city', *Medical History*, 32 (1988), 401–25.

27. Mary J. Dobson, *Contours of Death and Disease in Early Modern England* (Cambridge: Cambridge University Press, 1997) and John Landers, *Death and the Metropolis: Studies in the Demographic History of London, 1670–1830* (Cambridge: Cambridge University Press, 1993), 162–96.

28. The Meteorological Society was founded in 1850, the Association of Metropolitan Medical Officers of Health in 1856, and the Sanitary Institute in 1876.

29. The Liverpool story has been well covered by Paul Laxton and Gerry Kearns. See, in particular, Paul Laxton, 'Fighting for public health: Dr Duncan and his adversaries, 1847–63' in Sally Sheard and Helen Power (eds), *Body and City: Histories of Urban Public Health* (Aldershot: Ashgate, 2000), 59–88 and, in the same volume, Gerry Kearns, 'Town hall and Whitehall: sanitary intelligence in Liverpool, 1840–63', 89–108.

30. On the Metropolitan Asylums Board, see G.M. Ayers, *England's First State Hospitals and the Metropolitan Asylums Board, 1867–1930* (London: Wellcome Institute for the History of Medicine, 1967) and for the Registrar General's Office, John M. Eyler, *Victorian Social Medicine: The Ideas and Methods of William Farr* (Baltimore: Johns Hopkins University Press, 1979); Edward Higgs, *Life, Death and Statistics: Civil Registration, Censuses and the Work of the General Register Office* (Hatfield: Local Population Studies, 2004); and Libby Schweber, *Disciplining Statistics: Demography and Vital Statistics in France and England, 1830–1885* (London: Duke University Press, 2006), 93–130.

31. On medical officers' activities at local level Hardy, *Epidemic Streets* remains by far the best guide. See, also, the same author's summary account, 'Public health and the expert: the London medical officers of health, 1856–1900' in Roy MacLeod (ed.), *Government and Expertise: Specialists, Administrators and Professionals 1860– 1919* (Cambridge: Cambridge University Press, 1988), 128–44.

32. Gareth Stedman Jones, *Outcast London: A Study in the Relationship between Classes in Victorian Society* (Oxford: Oxford University Press, 1971), 159–238 and Anthony S. Wohl, *The Eternal Slum: Housing and Social Policy in Victorian London* (London: Edward Arnold, 1977), 26–39.

33. The central weakness of the large literature devoted to morbidity in the nineteenth century is that it has scarcely anything to say about unskilled, casual and workless labourers: there are no sources to help us recover and reconstruct the health biographies of these numerically overwhelmingly important categories. For more 'respectable' groups the work of James Riley has been preeminent – see, in particular, James C. Riley, *Sick Not Dead: The Health of British Workingmen during the Mortality Decline* (Baltimore: Johns Hopkins University Press, 1998). For an overview of the state of the art and an excellent bibliography see Bernard Harris, Martin Gorsky, Aravinda Guntupalli and Andrew Hinde, 'Ageing, sickness, and health in England and Wales during the mortality transition', *Social History of Medicine*, 24 (2011), 643–65.

34. For officially estimated rents among the poor and very poor in Hackney in north-east London see 'Report on the Housing of the Working Classes in Hackney', appended to *Hackney: Annual Report of the Medical Officer of Health 1901*.

35. By far the best account of metropolitan destitution and near-destitution remains Gareth Stedman Jones, *Outcast London*; but see also David Green, *From*

Artisans to Paupers: Economic Change and Poverty in London, 1790–1860 (Aldershot: Scolar Press, 1995).

36. In the capital these vast so-called 'pockets' of poverty became known as 'special areas', predictive of the officially designated 'depressed areas' of the interwar years. For a late nineteenth and early twentieth century metropolitan example see Graham Mooney and Andrea Tanner, 'Infant mortality, a spatial problem: Notting Dale special area' in Eilidh Garrett *et al.*, *Infant Mortality: A Continuing Social Problem* (Aldershot: Ashgate, 2006), 79–98.

37. The full emergence and development of the infant mortality debate and movement are discussed in Deborah Dwork, *War is Good for Babies and Other Young Children: A History of the Infant and Child Welfare Movement in England. 1898–1918* (London and New York: Tavistock Books, 1987); John M.Eyler, *Sir Arthur Newsholme and State Medicine 1885–1935* (Cambridge: Cambridge University Press, 1997), 295–340 and Garrett *et al.*, *Infant Mortality*.

38. Michael Worboys, *Spreading Germs: Disease Theories and Medical Practice in Britain 1865–1900* (Cambridge: Cambridge University Press, 2000), 126–9.

39. British Parliamentary Papers (BPP), *Royal Commission on Water Supply*, 1868–9, vol xxxiii., Q.3,906.

40. 'Jottings on the cholera', *Medical Times and Gazette*, ii, 1866, 174.

41. Ibid., 175

42. For the moral and social context see F.K. Prochaska, 'Philanthropy' in F.M.L. Thompson (ed.), *The Cambridge Social History of Britain: Volume 3 1750–1950* (Cambridge: Cambridge University Press, 1990), 357–94.

43. 'The cholera', *The Times*, 4 Aug. 1866.

44. Francis W. Sheppard, *London 1808–1870: The Infernal Wen* (London: Secker and Warburg, 1971), 274.

45. 'Jottings on the cholera', *Medical Press and Chronicle*, ii, 1866, 174–5.

46. *Sanitary Statistics and Proceedings: Bethnal Green: 1867*, 6.

47. See, in relation to the key indicator of infant mortality, Naomi Williams and Graham Mooney, 'Infant mortality in an "age of great cities": London and the provincial cities, c. 1850–1914', *Continuity and Change*, 9 (1994), 191–2. The typhoid index revealed much about adult well-being and, according to this measure, London was significantly healthier than the great majority of provincial cities with which it could be meaningfully compared. See Bill Luckin, *Pollution and Control: A Social History of the Thames in the Nineteenth Century* (Bristol and Boston: Adam Hilger, 1986), 123. Bristol had a better record than the capital and Birmingham and Bradford also performed well. At the bottom of the list, Salford recorded a typhoid death rate 70 per cent higher than London.

48. Derek Fraser, *Power and Authority in the Victorian City* (Oxford: Blackwell, 1979) set the pace. For a recent overview of comparative long-term differential urban political development see Ralf Roth and Robert Beachy (eds), *Who Ran the Cities: City Elites and Urban Power Structures in Europe and North America, 1750–1940* (Aldershot: Ashgate, 2007) and particularly, in that volume, James Moore

and Richard Rodger, 'Who really ran the cities? Municipal knowledge and policy networks in British local government, 1832–1914', 37–70.

49. On later nineteenth century Birmingham see E.P. Hennock, *Fit and Proper Persons: Ideal and Reality in Nineteenth Century Urban Government* (London: Edward Arnold, 1964). For Manchester see Harold L. Platt, *Shock Cities: The Environmental Transformation and Reform of Manchester and Chicago* (Chicago: University of Chicago Press, 2005), 313–32.

50. This intensely complicated issue has been expertly unravelled by John Davis in his *Reforming London: The London Government Problem 1855–1900* (Oxford: Clarendon Press, 1988). But see, also, David Owen, *The Government of Victorian London 1855–1889: The Metropolitan Board of Works, the Vestries and the City Corporation*, edited by Roy MacLeod (Cambridge Mass.: Harvard University Press, 1982).

51. For valuable contextual detail see D.H. Porter, *The Thames Embankment: Technology and Society in Victorian London* (Akron, Ohio: University of Akron Press, 1998). For the mid-century crisis, there is Steven Halliday, *The Great Stink of London: Sir Joseph Bazalgette and the Cleansing of the Victorian Metropolis* (Stroud: Sutton, 1998). See, also, for intriguing transcultural comparison, David S. Barnes, 'Confronting sensory crisis in the great stinks of London and Paris' in W.A. Cohen and Ryan Johnson (eds), *Filth: Dirt, Disgust and Modern Life* (Minneapolis: University of Minneapolis Press, 2005), 529–41.

52. The definitive account is Ken Young and Patricia L. Garside, *Metropolitan London: Politics and Urban Change 1837–1981* (London: Edward Arnold, 1982), chs 3 and 4. For up-to-date summaries of the peculiarities of the London government system at this time see also Jerry White, *London in the Nineteenth Century: 'A Human Awful Wonder of God'* (London: Vintage, 2008), 471–6 and Jerry White, *London in the Twentieth Century: A City and its People* (London: Vintage, 2001), 355–72.

53. See the still valuable W.W. Robson, *The Government and Misgovernment of London* (London: Allen and Unwin, 1939). In a splendidly biased onslaught, Robson attacks the performance of every metropolitan borough on one or many counts and makes a powerful early twentieth century plea for administrative centralization.

54. The literature here is large and diverse. See Joel A. Tarr, 'The metabolism of the industrial city: the case of Pittsburgh', *Journal of Urban History*, 28 (2002), 511–45: Christopher Hamlin, 'The city as a chemical system? The chemist as urban environmental professional in France and Britain 1780–1880', *Journal of Urban History*, 33 (2007), 702–28. See also the path-breaking Graeme Davison, 'The city as a natural system: theories of urban society in early nineteenth century Britain' in Derek Fraser and Anthony Sutcliffe (eds), *The Pursuit of Urban History* (London: Edward Arnold, 1983), 349–70.

55. See the important comparative study by Jamie Benidickson, *The Culture of Flushing: A Social and Legal History of Sewage* (Vancouver: University of British Columbia Press, 2007). Note, also, Daniel Schneider, *Hybrid Nature: Sewage*

Treatment and the Contradictions of the Industrial Ecosytem (Cambridge Mass.: MIT Press, 2011), 1–44.

56. Christopher Hamlin, *Public Health and Social Justice in the Age of Chadwick: Britain, 1800–1854* (Cambridge: Cambridge University Press, 1998), 16–51.

57. However, as Chapter 6 shows, the process could be astonishingly long drawn-out. As large towns and cities penetrated ever deeper into outer suburban and rural areas, and administratively colonized ever larger numbers of neighbouring communities, infrastructural systems rarely reached 'completion'.

58. See Tarr, 'The search for the ultimate sink: urban air, land and air pollution in historical perspective' in his *Ultimate Sink*, 7–35.

59. Historians are now digging deep into nineteenth century nuisances. See Chistopher Hamlin, 'Sanitary policing and the local state, 1873–74: a statistical study of English and Welsh towns', *Social History of Medicine*, 17 (2005), 39–61 and Hamlin, 'Public sphere to public health: the transformation of "nuisance"' in Steven Sturdy (ed.), *Medicine, Health and the Public Sphere in Britain, 1600–2000* (London: Routledge, 2002), 190–204. See, also, James G. Hanley, 'Parliament, physicians and nuisances: the demedicalization of nuisance law, 1831–1855', *Bulletin of the History of Medicine*, 80 (2006), 702–32 and Tom Crook, 'Sanitary inspection and the public sphere in late Victorian and Edwardian Britain: a case study in liberal governance', *Social History*, 32 (2007), 369–93.

60. Arguing that the idea reaches back to Hegel, William Cronon states that 'a kind of "second nature", designed by people and "improved" towards human ends, gradually emerged atop the landscape that nature – "first nature" – had created as such an inconvenient jumble'. Cronon, *Nature's Metropolis*, 56. My thanks to Rosalind Williams for guiding me to this reference.

61. On this overwhelmingly important nineteenth century ideology see Theodore K. Hoppen, *The Mid-Victorian Generation 1846–1886* (Oxford: Oxford University Press, 1998), 91–108 and the classic overview by Geoffrey Best in *Mid-Victorian Britain 1851–75* (London: Weidenfeld and Nicolson, 1971), 34–54. In the domain of health and environment see Christopher Hamlin, 'Muddling in bumbledom: on the enormity of large sanitary improvements in four British towns, 1855–1885', *Victorian Studies*, 32 (1988), 55–83.

62. There was no decisive and clear-cut moment at which distinctively environmental modes of thought became established. However, in terms of connections between the spread of infection and the variables that might determine that process, styles of thought, which break with sanitarianism, begin to establish themselves during the final 20 years of the nineteenth century. From the environmental perspective see Stephen Bocking, 'Environmentalism' in Peter L. Bowler and John V. Pickstone (eds), *The Cambridge History of Science. Volume Six. The Modern Biological and Earth Sciences* (Cambridge: Cambridge University Press, 2009), 602–21 and the invaluable James Winter, *Secure from Rash Assault: Sustaining the Victorian Environment*

(Berkeley: University of California Press, 1999). For changing and increasingly 'environmental' ways of conceptualizing germs, 'poison' and disease, there is Worboys, *Spreading Germs*.

63. See Bill Luckin, 'The shaping of a public environmental sphere in late nineteenth century London' in Sturdy, *Medicine, Health and the Public Sphere*, 229–34.

64. S.G. Checkland, *The Rise of Industrial Society in England 1815–1885* (London: Longmans, 1971), 170–1. The problem is also described by A.E. Dingle, '"The monster nuisance of all": landowners, alkali manufacturers and atmospheric pollution, 1828–64', *Economic History Review*, 35 (1982), 529–48.

65. However, Rollo Russell had been touched upon by Eric Ashby and Marion Anderson, *The Politics of Clean Air* (Oxford: Oxford University Press, 1981), 55–6 and Peter L.Brimblecombe, *The Big Smoke: A History of Air Pollution in London since Medieval Times* (London: Methuen, 1987), 109.

66. Very soon two excellent monographs appeared: Stephen Mosely, *The Chimney of the World: A History of Smoke Pollution in Victorian and Edwardian Manchester* (Cambridge: White Horse Press, 2001) and Peter Thorsheim, *Inventing Pollution: Coal Smoke and Culture in Britain since 1800* (Athens, OH: Ohio University Press, 2006). Thorsheim's primary focus is the capital.

67. Wood, *Demography of Victorian England and Wales*, 332–40 and 353.

68. For valuable biographical material on Rollo Russell see Philadelphia: American Philosophical Society Archive. 'Autobiographical note', B: R913 and Bertrand Russell and Patricia Russell (eds), *The Amberley Papers: Bertrand Russell's Family Background: Volume 2* (London: Hogarth Press, 1937), 532.

69. There is a large and multifaceted literature on urban degeneration. See in particular the pioneering Stedman Jones, *Outcast London*. See, also, Daniel Pick, *Faces of Degeneration: A European Disorder c. 1848–1918* (Cambridge: Cambridge University Press, 1989) and Jose Harris, *Private Lives and Public Spirit: Britain 1870–1914* (Oxford: Oxford University Press), 241–5. Bill Luckin, 'Revisiting the idea of urban degeneration in Victorian Britain', *Urban History*, 33 (2006), 234–52 covers the literature up until the early years of the new millennium.

70. W.S. Jevons, *The Coal Question: An Enquiry Concerning the Progress of the Nation* (Basingstoke: Palgrave, 2001). Reprint edition.

71. Patrick Brantlinger (ed.), *Energy and Entropy: Science and Culture in Victorian Britain: Essays from Victorian Studies* (Bloomington: Indiana University Press, 1989). See, also, Barri J. Gold, *Thermopoetics: Energy in Victorian Literature and Science* (Cambridge Mass.: MIT Press, 2010).

72. On Frankland see Colin A. Russell, *Edward Frankland: Chemistry, Controversy and Conspiracy in Victorian England* (Cambridge: Cambridge University Press, 1996). On Smith see Peter Reed, 'Robert Angus Smith and the Alkali Inspectorate' in E. Homburg, Anthony S. Travis and Harm G. Schroter (eds), *The Chemical Industry in Europe 1850–1914* (Dordrecht: Kluwer, 1998), 121–48 and Christine Garwood, 'Green crusaders or captives of industry? The

British Alkali industry and the ethics of environmental decision-making', *Annals of Science*, 61 (2004), 99–117.

73. Thorsheim, *Inventing Pollution*, 161–72 and Peter Thorsheim, 'Interpreting the London fog disaster of 1952' in E. Melanie Dupuis (ed.), *Smoke and Mirrors: The Politics and Culture of Air Pollution* (New York: New York University Press, 2004), 154–69.

74. For an overview see John A.Hassan, 'The water industry 1900–51: a failure of public policy?' in Robert Millward and John Singleton (eds), *The Political Economy of Nationalisation in Britain 1920–1950* (Cambridge: Cambridge University Press, 1995), 185–211.

75. From a demographic–epidemiological perspective Naomi Williams made a major contribution on the role and meanings of place and locality in 'Death in its season: class, environment and the mortality of infants in nineteenth century Sheffield', *Social History of Medicine*, 5 (1992), 71–94. The geographical and sociological literature is far too large to be meaningfully summarized.

76. Dolores Greenberg, 'Reconstructing race and protest: environmental justice in New York City', *Environmental History*, 5 (2000), 223–50.

77. H.L. Platt, 'Jane Addams and the ward boss revisited: class, politics and public health in Chicago, 1890–1930', *Environmental History*, 5 (2000), 194–222. See also the same author's *Shock Cities*, in which environmental justice is discussed at length.

78. The decisive studies of pollution in this context were Christopher Hamlin, *A Science of Impurity: Water Analysis in Nineteenth Century Britain* (Berkeley: University of California Press, 1990) and the same author's 'Environmental sensibility in Edinburgh, 1839–40: the "fetid irrigation" controversy', *Journal of Urban History*, 20 (1994), 311–39. See, also, for an important comparative perspective, Genevieve Massard-Guilbaud, *Histoire de la Pollution Industrielle: France 1789–1914* (Paris: Editions EHESS, 2010).

79. On the Victorian origins of environmental and ecological strands of thought see Peter L.Bowler, *The Norton History of the Environmental Sciences* (London: Norton, 1993) and James Winter, *Secure from Rash Assault*.

80. For 'second nature' see note 59 above.

81. Winter, *Secure from Rash Assault*, 19.

Chapter 2   Death and Survival in the City: Approaches to the History of Disease

1. A recent contributor to the debate qualifies what seem to be guardedly 'optimistic' conclusions by stating that 'the data on mortality rates in early nineteenth century cities seems damning enough, and I find myself in sympathy with the recent shift in emphasis to environmental factors'. G. N. Von

Tunzelmann. 'Trends in real wages, 1750–1850, revisited', *Economic History Review*, xxxii (1979), 49.

2. Michel Foucault, *The Birth of the Clinic: An Archaeology of Medical Perception* (London: Tavistock, 1973). Translated by A. M. Sheridan. See also Brian Abel-Smith, *The Hospitals, 1800–1948: A Study in Social Administration in England and Wales* (London: Heinemann, 1964).

3. The classical journal is Erwin H. Ackerknecht, 'Anticontagionism between 1821 and 1867', *Bulletin of the History of Medicine*, xxii (1948), 562–93.

4. See, for example, George Rosen, *A History of Public Health* (New York: MD Publications, 1958) and 'Disease, debility and death' in H. J. Dyos and Michael Wolff (eds), *The Victorian City: Images and Realities, Volume 2* (London: Routledge and Kegan Paul, 1973), 625–67.

5. For a typically dazzling and deeply considered synopsis see Joseph Needham (with Lu Gwei-Djen), 'Medicine and Chinese culture' in Joseph Needham, *Clerks and Craftsmen in China and the West* (Cambridge: Cambridge University Press, 1970), 263–93.

6. Carlo M. Cipolla, *Cristofano and the Plague: A Study in the History of Public Health in the Age of Galileo* (London: Collins, 1973) and Cipolla, *Public Health and the Medical Profession in the Renaissance* (Cambridge: Cambridge University Press, 1976).

7. Keith Thomas, *Religion and the Decline of Magic: Studies in Popular Beliefs in Sixteenth and Seventeenth Century England* (London: Weidenfeld and Nicolson, 1973), 209–52. However, the social and sociological frameworks within which historians might more fruitfully examine interactions between 'specialist' and 'non-specialist' world-views have only recently begun to be discussed. For a brave venture in this field see Janet Blackman, 'Popular theories of generation: the evolution of *Aristotle's Works*. The study of an anachronism', in John Woodward and David Richards (eds), *Health Care and Popular Medicine in Nineteenth Century England* (London: Croom Helm, 1977), 56–89.

8. Andrew B. Appleby, 'Disease or famine? Mortality in Cumberland and Westmorland 1580–1640', *Economic History Review*, xxvi (1973), 403–33 and the same author's 'Nutrition and disease: the case of London, 1550–1750', *Journal of Interdisciplinary History*, vi (1975), 1–22.

9. Ivan Illich, *Limits to Medicine: Medical Nemesis* (London: Calder and Boyars,1977); Philipe Aries, *Western Attitudes Towards Death: From the Middle Ages to the Present* (Baltimore: Johns Hopkins University Press, 1974). Illich's study contains a superlative bibliography on the history and sociology of medicine and disease.

10. S. E. Finer, *The Life and Times of Sir Edwin Chadwick* (London: Methuen, 1952): R. A. Lewis, *Edwin Chadwick and the Public Health Movement 1832–1854* (London: Longmans, Green, 1952):R. S. Lambert, *Sir John Simon 1816–1904 and English Social Administration* (London: MacGibbon and Kee, 1963). These seminal studies have now been complemented by Margaret Pelling's scholarly

account of medical and epidemiological thought, *Cholera, Fever and the English Medicine 1825–1865* (Oxford: Oxford University Press, 1978).

11. Exceptions include Peter Razzell, *The Conquest of Smallpox: The Impact of Inoculation on Smallpox Mortality in Eighteenth Century Britain* (Firle, Sussex: Caliban Books, 1977) and Alan Armstrong, *Stability and Change in an English County Town: A Social Study of York 1801–1851* (Cambridge: Cambridge University Press, 1974), 108–54.

12. The arguments contained in these journals have now been restated and expanded in Thomas McKeown, *The Modern Rise of Population* (London: Edward Arnold, 1976).

13. Charles Murchison, *The Continued Fevers of Great Britain* (London, 1884, 3rd edition), 52–3: *Report of the Medical Officer of Health: Shoreditch 1862*, 19: *Report of the Medical Officer of Health: Strand 1859*, 11: and *Report of the Medical Officer of Health: Holborn 1866*, 53–4.

14. Admissions material for London for the period 1848–70 is to be found in Murchison, *Continued Fevers*, 74–5. Data for the final 30 years of the century may be abstracted from the *Minutes* of the Metropolitan Asylums Board and, from 1887 onwards, from the annual *Reports* of the Board's Statistical Committee.

15. Local differentials in levels of rent have not yet been studied in depth but there is much relevant and penetrating material in E. H. Hunt, *Regional Wage Variations in Britain 1850–1914* (Oxford: Oxford University Press, 1973). On dietary history see Derek Oddy and Derek Miller (eds), *The Making of the Modern British Diet* (London: Croom Helm, 1976) and the trenchant remarks in F. B. Smith, *The People's Health 1830–1910* (London: Weidenfeld and Nicolson, 1979). The interpretative historical literature in English on this topic is still underdeveloped. For recent work in French, much of it influenced by the *Annales* school, see Illich, *Medical Nemesis*.

16. On the Thames question at this time see *Royal Commission on the Supply of Water in the Metropolis*, British Parliamentary Papers (BPP), 1828, vol. ix., 122–3 and 200. On St Helens, see S. G. Checkland, *The Rise of Industrial Society in England 1815–1885* (London: Longmans, 1971), 170–1.

17. The most important pioneer in the field of applied water analysis was the chemist, Edward Frankland. For a brief biographical note see J. R. Partington, *A History of Chemistry, Volume 4* (London: Macmillan,1964), 500–1. The crucial figure in the development of the monitoring of atmospheric pollution was the influential Angus Smith. See Roy M. MacLeod, 'The Alkali Acts Administration 1863–84: the emergence of the civil scientist', *Victorian Studies*, ix (1965), 85–112.

18. This topic has been discussed by, among others, Gareth Stedman Jones, *Outcast London: A Study of the Relationship between Classes in Victorian Society* (Oxford: Oxford University Press, 1971) and A. S. Wohl, *The Eternal Slum: Housing and Social Policy in Victorian London* (London: Edward Arnold, 1977). See also S. D.

Chapman (ed.), *The History of Working Class Housing: A Symposium* (Newton Abbot: David and Charles, 1971).

19. Information of this kind is available for the London Fever Hospital and for institutions which came under the jurisdiction of the Metropolitan Asylums Board.

20. See note 15 above.

21. John C. Synder, 'The typhus fevers' in Thomas M. Rivers (ed.), *Viral and Rickettsial Infections of Man* (Philadelphia: J.B. Lippincott, 1952), 578–610, and Thomas McKeown, R. G. Brown and R. G. Record, 'An interpretation of the modern rise of population in Europe', *Population Studies*, xxvi (1972), 345–82 and, particularly, 356.

22. The general 'hygiene' argument has been put forward by P. E. Razzell, 'An interpretation of the modern rise of population in Europe – a critique', *Population Studies*, xxviii (1974), 5–17. On typhus see J. D. Chambers, *Population, Economy and Society in Pre-Industrial England* (Oxford: Oxford University Press, 1972), 103–4.

23. This is the general explanation proposed by McKeown, *Modern Rise of Population*. But note the suggestive qualifications proposed by Robert Woods, 'Mortality and sanitary conditions in the "best governed city in the world" – Birmingham, 1870–1910', *Journal of Historical Geography*, iv (1978), 35–56.

24. George Rosen, 'Disease, debility and death', 650.

25. Fernand Braudel, *Capitalism and Material Life* (London: Weidenfeld and Nicolson, 1974). Translated by Miriam Kochan: Louis Henry, 'The population of France in the eighteenth century', in D. V. Glass and David Eversley (eds), *Population in History* (London: Edward Arnold, 1965), 448: Chambers, *Population, Economy and Society*, ch. 4. The subject is also clearly examined in John D. Post, 'Famine, mortality and epidemic disease in the process of modernization', *Economic History Review*, xxix (1976), 14–38. There is much that is germane to this topic in William H. McNeill, *Plagues and Peoples* (Oxford: Blackwell, 1977), an ambitious interpretation of ecological history, based on wide-ranging medico-historical documentation.

26. Macfarlane Burnet and David O. White, *The Natural History of Infectious Disease* (Cambridge: Cambridge University Press, 1972).

27. Paul Slack, 'Disease and the social historian', *Times Literary Supplement*, 8 March 1974.

28. T. S. McKeown and R. G. Record, 'Reasons for the decline of mortality in England and Wales during the nineteenth century', *Population Studies*, xvi (1962), 94–122, reprinted in M. W. Flinn and T. C. Smout (eds), *Essays in Social History* (Oxford: Clarendon Press Press, 1974), 218–55. Scarlet fever is discussed at several points in this influential article but see, in particular, p. 243.

29. In the period between about 1830 and 1900 case fatality rates ranged fairly consistently between 25 and 40 per cent. *Fifth Annual Report of the Poor Law Commission*, BPP, 1839, vol. xx, Appendix C2, 113: annual *Reports* of the Statistical Committee of the Metropolitan Asylums Board 1887–1900: E. W.

Goodall, *A Short History of the Infectious Epidemic Diseases* (London: John Bale, 1934), 88.

30. Asa Briggs, 'Cholera and society in the nineteenth century', *Past and Present*, 19 (1961), 79–96.

31. Popular hostility towards the medical profession is well described by Michael Durey, *The First Spasmodic Cholera Epidemic in York, 1832*. (York: Borthwick Papers, no. 46, 1974).

32. The literature is now becoming voluminous. A basic bibliography, excluding unpublished Ph.D and M. A. theses, would include R. E. McGraw, *Russia and the Cholera 1823–32* (Madison: University of Wisconsin Press, 1965): Louis Chevalier (ed.), *Le Choléra: La Premiére Epidémie du XIXe siècle* (La Roche-sur-Yon, 1958); Charles Rosenberg, *The Cholera Years: The United States in 1832, 1849 and 1866* (Chicago: University of Chicago Press, 1962); R. J. Morris, *Cholera 1832: The Social Response to an Epidemic* (London: Croom Helm, 1976). A more exhaustive bibliography is contained in Pelling, *Cholera and English Fever*.

33. The Society for the Social History of Medicine provides a stimulating point of contact for those engaged on research in this field. Its journal, the *Bulletin of the Society for the Social History of Medicine*, contains regular summaries of work in progress.

Chapter 3   Evaluating the Sanitary Revolution: Typhus and Typhoid in London, 1851–1900

1. For a classic 'biography' of typhus by a great medical scientist see Hans Zinsser, *Rats, Lice and History* (London: George Routledge,1935). There is also valuable information in K. F. Helleiner, 'The population of Europe from the Black Death to the eve of the vital revolution', *Cambridge Economic History of Europe: Volume Four* (Cambridge: Cambridge University Press, 1967), 1–95: Charles Creighton, *A History of Epidemics in Britain, Volume 2* (London: Cass, 1965), edited by David Eversley. See also J. D. Chambers, *Population, Economy and Society in Pre-Industrial England* (Oxford: Oxford University Press, 1972). There is no comparable secondary work on typhoid but the reader can derive a basic framework from Creighton.

2. M. W. Flinn, 'The stabilization of mortality in pre-industrial Europe', *Journal of European Economic History*, 3 (1974), 285–318 and *idem*, 'Plague in Europe and the Mediterranean countries', *Journal of European Economic History*, 8 (1979), 131–48.

3. Michel Foucault dominates the historiography in this field. See, in particular, *The Birth of the Clinic: An Archaeology of Medical Perception* (London: Tavistock, 1973). Translated by A. M. Sheridan. On asylums and prisons in Britain see Andrew Scull, *Museums of Madness: The Social Origins of Insanity in Nineteenth-Century England* (London: Allen Lane, 1979) and Michael Ignatieff, *A Just*

Measure of Pain: The Penitentiary in the Industrial Revolution, 1750–1850 (London: Macmillan, 1978).

4. There are no systematic studies of the impact of typhoid on urban or rural communities during the late eighteenth and early nineteenth centuries. But one notorious 'closed community', Millbank Prison, was repeatedly afflicted during the early nineteenth century. For a full and revealing account see British Parliamentary Papers (BPP), *Rivers Pollution Commissioners, Sixth Report: Domestic Water Supply of Great Britain,* 1874, vol. xxxiii, 165–6 and 495.

5. Creighton, *History of Epidemics*, 160 passim.

6. The demographic dimension is clearly set out in Thomas McKeown, *The Modern Rise of Population* (London: Edward Arnold, 1976).

7. Medical information on typhus has been drawn principally from E. S. Murphy, 'Typhus fever group'in P. D. Hoeprich (ed.), *Infectious Diseases* (London: Harper and Row, 1972), 791–9 and J. C. Snyder, 'The typhus fevers'in T. M. Rivers (ed.), *Viral and Rickettsial Infections of Man* (Philadelphia: J.B. Lippincott,1952), 578–610.

8. This estimate is based on E. W. Goodall, *A Short History of the Infectious Epidemic Diseases* (London, John Bale, 1934), 88; BPP, *Fifth Annual Report of the Poor Law Commission,* 1839, vol. xx, Appendix C2, 113: *Minutes,* Metropolitan Asylums Board, 2 Nov. 1872, 408–9: and *Minutes,* Association of Medical Officers of Health, 19 March 1864.

9. Medical material on typhoid has been derived from F. S. Stewart, *Bigger's Handbook of Bacteriology* (London: Balliere, Tindall and Cassell, 1962), 328–50 and A. Patrick, *The Enteric Fevers* (Edinburgh: Royal College of Physicians of Edinburgh Publications no. 2, 1955).

10. This estimate is based on data in the unnumbered pull-out tables in the *Annual Reports* of the Statistical Committee of the Metropolitan Asylums Board between 1890 and 1902; *Report of the Medical Officer of Health to the London County Council, 1910,* 44; and Charles Murchison, *A Treatise on the Continued Fevers of Great Britain* (London, 1884, 3rd edition), 604.

11. R. Thorne, *The Progress of Medicine During the Victorian Era, 1837–87* (London: Shaw, 1888), 26.

12. G. B. Longstaff, 'The seasonal prevalence of continued fever in London', *Transactions of the Epidemiological Society of London* (1884–5), 72, and Murchison, *Continued Fevers* (1873, 2nd edition), 682.

13. J. N. Radcliffe, 'Reports on epidemics', *Transactions of the Epidemiological Society of London* (1863), 411 and Creighton, *History of Epidemics*, 201.

14. Murchison, *Continued Fevers* (1884, 3rd edition), 52

15. *Minutes of Committees,* Metropolitan Asylums Board, 6 Nov. 1869 and 23 April 1870.

16. *Report of the MOH: Hackney 1864,* 13 and *Hackney: Report 1878,* 4; A. Hill, 'Diphtheria and typhoid and their concomitant conditions in Birmingham', *Transactions of the Society of Medical Officers of Health* (1879–80), 70.

17. *Report of the MOH: Shoreditch 1862,* 19; *Report of the MOH: Strand 1859,* 11; and *Report of the MOH: Holborn 1866,* 53–4.

18. Major Greenwood, *Epidemics and Crowd Diseases* (London: Williams and Norgate, 1935), 158.

19. Metropolitan Association of Medical Officers of Health, *Memorandum concerning the Present Prevalence of Typhus Fever in London,* 21 Nov. 1863; *Report of the MOH: Whitechapel, First Quarter, 1862,* 5; *Report of the MOH: Shoreditch, 1862,* 19–20.

20. Creighton, *History of Epidemics,* 215.

21. G. Rosen, 'Disease, debility and death', in H. J. Dyos and Michael Wolff (eds), *The Victorian City: Volume 2* (London: Routledge and Kegan Paul, 1973), 633–4; and Rosen, *A History of Public Health* (New York: MD Publications, 1958), 339–40.

22. T. McKeown and R. G. Record, 'Reasons for the decline of mortality in England and Wales during the nineteenth century', *Population Studies,* 16 (1962), 94–122.

23. W. R. Baldwin-Wiseman, 'The increase in the national consumption of water', *Journal of the Royal Statistical Society,* 122 (1909), 282–90.

24. Ibid., 282.

25. This calculation is based on data in BPP, *Rivers Pollution Commissioners, Sixth Report,* 622: *Report of Epidemic Cholera in England 1866,* 1867–8, vol. xxxvii, 374 and Table 33; *Report of the General Board of Health on the Supply of Water to the Metropolis,* 1850, vol. xxii, 6: and population statistics in the relevant *Annual* and *Supplementary Reports* of the Registrar- General.

26. *Royal Commission on the Water Supply of the Metropolis,* 1893–4, 16: *Report of the Medical Officer of Health to the London County Council, 1892,* 42.

27. For a comparative statement of the work completed at district level see BPP. *Metropolitan Sanitary and Street Improvements,* 1872, vol. xlix, 585–654.

28. Baldwin-Wiseman, 'National consumption of water'.

29. An environmental process of this kind was perceptively identified by W. D. Scott-Moncrieff, 'River pollution: its ethics, aesthetics and hygiene', *Journal of the Royal Sanitary Institute* 30 (1909), 165–72.

30. The connection between overcrowding and typhus was noted by numerous contemporary medical men. See, for example, *Report of the MOH: Bethnal Green, 1864,* 4; *Report of the MOH: St George-in-the-East, 1865,* 27; and *idem,* 1868, 19. The literature by historians emphasizing the 'crisis of the inner city' in the 1860s, and thereafter, includes Gareth Stedman Jones, *Outcast London: A Study in the Relationship between Classes in Victorian Society* (Oxford: Oxford University Press, 1971), Part 2: H. J. Dyos, 'Railways and housing in Victorian London', *Journal of Transport History,* 2 (1955), 11–21 and, 'Some social costs of railway building in London', *Journal of Transport History* 3 (1957–8), 23–30. Housing indices have been authoritatively examined by A. S. Wohl, 'The housing of the working classes in London, 1815–1914' in S. D. Chapman (ed.), *The History of Working-Class Housing: A Symposium* (Newton Abbott: David and Charles,

1971), 15-54 and *The Eternal Slum: Housing and Social Policy in Victorian London* (London: Edward Arnold, 1977).

31. *Minutes,* Metropolitan Association of Medical Officers of Health, 19 March 1864: *Report of the MOH: Whitechapel: Second Quarter, 1862,* 5; and *Whitechapel, Report Quarter ending 28th. December 1867,* 8.

32. S. B. Saul, *The Myth of the Great Depression* (London: Macmillan, 1969), 30-4.

33. See the cautious assessments of J. C. Snyder, 'Typhus fevers', 596; A. B. Appleby, 'Nutrition and disease: the case of London, 1550-1750', *Journal of Interdisciplinary History* 6 (1975), 2 and 13; and T. McKeown, R. G. Brown and R. G. Record, 'An interpretation of the modern rise of population in Europe', *Population Studies,* 26 (1972), 356.

34. A means of testing such an association is available in the table of London bread prices compiled by B. R. Mitchell and P. Deane, *Abstract of British Historical Statistics* (Cambridge: Cambridge University Press, 1962), 497-8.

35. The statistical information for Scotland needs separate consideration.

36. McKeown and Record, 'Reasons for the decline of mortality', 120-1.

37. There is no evidence to suggest that there was any development of the milder, endemic Brill-Zinsser variant identified among immigrants to the United States. From a now large literature see the pioneering Hans Zinsser, 'Varieties of typhus virus and the epidemiology of the American form of European typhus fever (Brill's disease)', *American Journal of Hygiene,* 20 (1934), 513-32.

38. For a stimulating analysis of theoretically possible modifications for a different infection see A. B. Appleby, 'The disappearance of the plague', *Economic History Review,* 33 (1980), 161-73.

39. On the general topic of typhus and migration see J. W. D. Megaw, 'Typhus fevers and other rickettsial fevers' in *The British Encyclopaedia of Medical Practice, Volume 2* (London: Butterworth, 1952), 393. For London see *Report of the MOH: Mile End Old Town, 1861,* 6. For relatively high and continuing rates of migration from Ireland to the north-west and the north-east during this period see Creighton, *History of Epidemics,* 215-17 and J. W. House, *North Eastern England: Population Movements and the Landscape since the early Nineteenth Century* (Durham: University of Durham, King's College Department of Geography Research Series no. 1,1954), 51-62.

40. Brinley Thomas, *Migration and Economic Growth: Great Britain and the Atlantic Economy* (Cambridge: Cambridge University Press, 1954), 73.

41. L. H. Lees, *Exiles of Erin: Irish Migrants in Victorian London* (Manchester: Manchester University Press, 1979), 47. Some of these arguments are also examined in the American context in R. Higgs, 'Cycles and trends in mortality in 18 large American cities, 1871-1900', *Explorations in Economic History,* 16 (1979), 381-408.

42. The general epidemiological context has been meticulously described by Margaret Pelling, *Cholera, Fever and English Medicine, 1825-1865* (Oxford:

Oxford University Press, 1978). Accounts of specific typhoid outbreaks are to be found in *Report of the MOH: Kensington, 1873,* 69–70; *Report of the MOH: Hackney, 1882,* 6; and *Report of the MOH: St Pancras, 1891,* 17–18.

43. On milk transmission see G. P. Gladstone, 'Pathogenicity and virulence of microorganisms', in Howard Florey (ed.), *General Pathology* (London: Lloyd-Luke, 1970), 840, and J. Ritchie, 'Enteric fever', *British Medical Journal,* ii (1937), 166. Important milk-borne epidemics in the capital are described in BPP. *Supplementary Report of the Medical Officer to the Privy Council and Local Government Board,* 1874, vol. xxxi, Appendix 6: *Report of the MOH: St Pancras, 1883,* 15–18 and *Report of the MOH: Islington, 1883,* 54–6.

44. See Arthur Newsholme, *Fifty Years in Public Health* (London: Allen and Unwin,1935), 205–6: *Report of the MOH: Lambeth, 1894,* 4–36; *Report of the MOH: Fulham, 1899,* 18–19; and *Report of the MOH: St Pancras, 1900,* 39–41.

45. The discovery is usually attributed to Karl Wilhelm Drigalski in 1903. See Charles Singer and E. A. Underwood, *A Short History of Medicine* (Oxford: Clarendon Press, 1962), 407–9.

46. *RC Water Supply of the Metropolis,* Appendix C 17, 220 and 227.

47. Ibid., 224.

48. For the continuing phenomenon of small-scale outbreaks in middle-class homes compare *Report of the MOH: Hackney, 1862,* 13–14 and *Report of the MOH: St George, Hanover Square, 1890,* 109–10.

49. This figure has been computed from data contained in the tables of the *Annual Reports* of the Statistical Committee of the Metropolitan Asylums Board from 1890 to 1902. Aggregate statistics from this source have been checked against returns in the *Annual Reports* of the Registrar-General.

50. G. M. Ayers, *England's First State Hospitals and the Metropolitan Asylums Board, 1867–1930* (London: Wellcome Institute for the History of Medicine, 1971), 89–90.

51. The case rate per thousand of population in London declined from 0.78 in 1891–95 to 0.52 in 1901–05. See S. Davies,' Twenty years' advance in preventative medicine', *Public Health,* 21 (1908), 116. For a similar interpretation see Ayers, *England's First State Hospitals,* 106.

52. *Report of the MOH: St Giles, 1898–9,* 101–4. On occasion, however, vestries could be penny-pinching in their attitude towards this novel institution. See *St Luke Vestry: Annual Report: 1899,* 63.

53. Frankland was repeatedly assailed by a group of chemists and public health specialists, who were generally sympathetic towards the water companies, and who disagreed with his methodology for assessing the safety or otherwise of drinking water. The most persistent protagonists were Henry Letheby, J. A. Wanklyn and C. M. Tidy. From a wide-ranging and important literature see *RC Water Supply, Minutes of Evidence,* 1868–9, qs. 5418–22; *Select Committee on Metropolitan Water Supply (No. 2),* 1871, vol. xi, q. 1,277; and *Minutes,* Metropolitan Association of Medical Officers of Health, 18 Jan. 1878.

54. See, for example, his 'over-cautious' evidence to the *RC Water Supply, Minutes of Evidence,* 1868–9, qs. 6,401 and 6,418 and *Rivers Pollution Commission: Sixth Report,* 768.

55. On the influence of the Metropolitan Association of Medical Officers of Health see *Public Health: Jubilee Number* (1906) and A. S. Wohl, 'Unfit for human habitation' in Dyos and Wolff, *Victorian City: Volume 2,* 603–24.

56. One informal means of contact may have been the 'X' Club of which Frankland was a prominent member. See R. M. Macleod, 'The X-Club: a social network of science in Victorian England', *Notes and Records of the Royal Society,* 24 (1970), 305–22 and J. Vernon Jenson, 'The X-Club: a fraternity of Victorian scientists', *British Journal for the History of Science,* 5 (1970–1), 63–72. The pivotal importance of William Farr has recently been explored in J. M. Eyler, *Victorian Social Medicine: The Ideas and Methods of William Farr* (Baltimore: Johns Hopkins University Press, 1979).

Chapter 4   The Final Catastrophe: Cholera in London, 1866

1. On no day between 21 July and 6 August did fewer than a hundred inhabitants in the East End perish from the disease: and only at the beginning of November did weekly fatalities decline to approximately 20. See 'Mr J. Netten Radcliffe on cholera in London, and especially the eastern districts' in *Ninth Report of the Medical Officer of the Privy Council,* British Parliamentary Papers (BPP) 1867, vol. xxxvii, Appendix 7, Tables vi, vii and viii.

2. A basic chronology of the epidemic and its alleged determinants may be derived from Norman Longmate, *King Cholera* (London: Hamish Hamilton, 1966), 212–22. Francis W. Sheppard, *London 1808–1870: The Infernal Wen* (London: Secker and Warburg, 1971), 294–6; Henry Jephson, *The Sanitary Evolution of London* (London: T. Fisher Unwin, 1907), 189–92 and William A. Robson, *The Government and Misgovernment of London* (London: Allen and Unwin, 1948), 105–6.

3. On historical methodologies for assessing the extent and duration of water-borne epidemics see M. Durey, *The First Spasmodic Cholera Epidemic in York* (York: St Anthony's Press, 1974), 9–12.

4. This, and subsequent letters are reprinted in *Report of Epidemic Cholera in England 1866,* BPP, 1867–8, vol. xxxvii, 191.

5. Farr to Frankland, 31 July 1866.

6. *The Times,* 2 Aug. 1866.

7. Jephson, *Sanitary Evolution,* 191.

8. *The Times,* 2 Aug. 1866.

9. Farr to Valentin, 3 Aug. 1866.

10. *Report of Epidemic Cholera 1866,* 229.

11. *Report of Captain Tyler to the Board of Trade in regard to the East London Waterworks Company,* BPP, 1867, vol. lviii, 444. Evidence of Dr Corner.

12. The principal tenets of the doctrine are set out in *Report of the Medical Council in Relation to the Cholera Epidemic of 1854*, BPP, 1854–5, vol. xlv, 6; and *Report of the Committee for Scientific Inquiries in Relation to the Cholera Epidemic of 1854*, BPP, 1854–5, vol. xxi, 51. See also, William Farr, 'The cholera epidemic of 1853–4' in *Seventeenth Annual Report of the Registrar-General*, 74–108.

13. *Report of Epidemic Cholera 1866*, 278. Evidence of Henry N. Pink.

14. *Report of the Medical Officer of Health: Bethnal Green: 1866*, 20.

15. For a concise delineation of Pettenkofer's work see Major Greenwood, *Epidemics and Crowd Diseases* (London: Williams and Norgate, 1935), 150–9.

16. *Report of Epidemic Cholera 1866*, 263. Evidence of F. Godrich.

17. Orton's views on the epidemic are contained in two pungent reports. 'Special Report by Thomas Orton, Medical Officer of Health, Limehouse, on the Cholera Epidemic of 1866' (London, 1866); and *Report of the Medical Officer of Health Limehouse (1867) with Supplementary and Conclusive Remarks on the Cholera Epidemic in East London*. Orton was particularly scathing towards Captain Tyler, the Board of Trade inspector, whose training, like so many public health functionaries of the time, had been military rather than medical. See Orton, 'Special Report', 13.

18. Orton, 'Special Report', 4.

19. Orton, *Report 1867*, 10.

20. Snow's classic formulation had been: 'I consider that the cause of cholera is always cholera; that each case always depends upon a previous one', *Select Committee on Public Health and Nuisances Removal Bill*, BPP, 1854–5, vol. xiii, q. 150. There are interesting parallels with attitudes towards cholera transmission discerned among American doctors and sanitarians by Charles Rosenberg, *The Cholera Years: The United States in 1832, 1849 and 1866* (Chicago: University of Chicago Press, 1962), 199. On this broader issue of the acceptance or rejection of the germ theory see E. H. Ackerknecht, 'Anticontagionism between 1821 and 1867', *Bulletin of the History of Medicine*, 22, 1948, 562–93; and J. K. Crellin, 'The dawn of the germ theory: particles, infection and biology' in F. N. L. Poynter (ed.), *Science and Medicine in the 1860s* (London: Wellcome Institute of the History of Medicine, 1968), 57–76.

21. The policy of the water companies at this time is summarized in Robson, *Government and Misgovernment*, 100–120. See also, A. K. Mukhopadhyay, 'Politics of London water supply 1871–1971', Ph.D. thesis, University of London, 1972.

22. For contemporary examples of 'domestic pollution' see *Report of the Medical Officer of Health: Shoreditch 1859*, 12–13: and *Report of the Medical Officer of Health: Hackney, 1862*, 13–14.

23. See, for example, the comments on this topic in *Eleventh Report of the Medical Officer of Health: Mile End Old Town*, 17: and *Rivers Pollution Commissioners: Second Report: River Lea*, BPP 1867, vol. xxxvii, q. 3, 220. Evidence of James Knight, surveyor to the vestry of Mile End Old Town.

24. This compromise position is well demonstrated by the remarks of J. J. Rygate in *Eleventh Report of the Medical Officer of Health: St. George-in-the-East*, 26–7.

25. Letheby tended to take up a sanguine attitude towards the quality of the capital's water supply, and he thus frequently crossed swords with the more sceptical Edward Frankland. See, for example, Letheby's remarks to the Metropolitan Association of Medical Officers of Health: *Minutes: Ordinary Meetings*, 17 April and 1 May 1869.

26. *Tyler's Report*, 460.

27. *Select Committee on the East London Water Bills*, BPP, 1867, vol. ix, 363.

28. *Royal Commission on Water Supply*, BPP, 1868–9, vol. xxxiii, q. 3, 906.

29. *Tyler's Report*, 458–9.

30. *Rivers Pollution Commissioners: Lea*, q. 203.

31. *Tyler's Report*, 448.

32. Ibid., 460.

33. *Rivers Pollution Commissioners: Lea*, xxi.

34. *The Lancet*, 2 Nov. 1867.

35. *SC East London Water Bills*, xiii.

36. 'Copy of Correspondence between the Board of Trade and the East London Waterworks Company with Reference to Captain Tyler's Report on the Water Supplied by the Company', BPP, 1867, vol. lviii, 481–93.

37. Ibid., 486.

38. Ibid., 490–3.

39. *Report of Epidemic Cholera 1866*, xliv.

40. *British Medical Journal*, 16 Nov. 1867.

41. *The Lancet*, 2 Nov. 1867.

42. *RC Water Supply*, q. 7,127.

43. 'Radcliffe on cholera', 368.

44. R. S. Lambert, *Sir John Simon 1816–1904 and English Social Administration* (London: MacGibbon and Kee, 1963), part iv, *passim*.

45. *Twelfth Report of the Medical Officer of the Privy Council*, BPP, 1870, vol. xxxviii, 611.

46. 'Radcliffe on cholera', 331.

47. See the definitive analysis in R. A. Lewis, *Edwin Chadwick and the Public Health Movement 1832–1854* (London: Longmans Green, 1952), 258–79.

48. For a penetrating interpretation of the wider impact of the ideas of the two innovators see Margaret Pelling, 'Some approaches to nineteenth century epidemiology with particular reference to John Snow and William Budd', B. Litt. Thesis, University of Oxford, 1971.

49. Material on popular attitudes to polluted water may be found in *Report of the General Board of Health on Epidemic Cholera*, BPP, 1851, vol. xxi, 21. Evidence of Dr Gavin, *Report of the General Board of Health on the Supply of Water to the Metropolis*, BPP, 1850, xxii, qs. 724–31. Evidence of Robert Bowie and Dr Gavin; and *Select Committee on the Metropolis Water Bill*, BPP, 1851, vol. xv, q. 6,139.

50. On the theoretical content of Farr's approach see John M. Eyler: 'William Farr on the cholera: the sanitarian's disease theory and the statistician's method', *Journal of the History of Medicine and Allied Sciences*, 28 (1973), 79–100.

51. Edward Frankland's role during this period was of central importance. Despite his continuingly informal and advisory status in the 20 years following the epidemic, he successfully extended and elaborated his analytical methodology. An impression of his dynamic conception of the water problem may be gained by comparing his early comments in *Report* in BPP, 1872, vol. xlix, 804–8, with his mature *Report* for 1891 in *Registrar-General: Summary* 1890–1, xliii–lii.

Chapter 5   The Metropolitan and the Municipal: The Politics of Health and Environment, 1860–1920

1. David Reeder, 'Conclusions: perspectives on metropolitan administrative history' in David Owen, *The Government of Victorian London 1855–1889: The Metropolitan Board of Works, the Vestries and the City Corporation*, edited by Roy MacLeod (London: Harvard University Press, 1982), 349.

2. Christopher Hamlin, 'Edward Frankland's early career as London's official water analyst, 1865–1876: the context of "previous sewage contamination"', *Bulletin of the History of Medicine*, 56 (1982), 56–76 and the same author's *A Science of Impurity: Water Analysis in Nineteenth Century Britain* (Berkeley: University of California Press, 1990).

3. The full range of arguments is surveyed in John Davis, *Reforming London: The London Government Problem, 1855–1900* (Oxford: Clarendon Press, 1988). See also Ken Young and Patricia L. Garside, *Metropolitan London: Politics and Urban Change, 1837–1981* (London: Edward Arnold, 1982). Other excellent overviews include P.J. Waller, *Town, City and Nation: England 1850–1914* (Oxford: Oxford University Press, 1983), 24–67; Patricia L. Garside, 'London and the Home Counties' in F.M.L. Thompson (ed.), *Cambridge Social History of Britain, Volume 1: Regions and Communities* (Cambridge: Cambridge University Press, 1990), 471–539; Richard Dennis, 'Modern London' in M. Daunton (ed.), *Cambridge Urban History of Britain Volume 3: 1840–1950* (Cambridge: Cambridge University Press, 2000), 95–132 and Asa Briggs's seminal *Victorian Cities* (London: Odham's Press, 1963), 311–60.

4. John Landers, *Death and the Metropolis: Studies in the Demographic History of London 1670–1830* (Cambridge: Cambridge University Press, 1993). See also L.D. Schwarz, *London in the Age of Industrialization: Entrepreneurs, Labour Force and Living Conditions, 1700–1850* (Cambridge: Cambridge University Press, 1992), part 2 and the same author's 'London 1700–1840' in P. Clark (ed.), *Cambridge Urban History of Britain Volume 2: 1540–1840* (Cambridge: Cambridge University Press, 2000), 649–55.

5. Roderick Floud, Kenneth Wachter and Annabel Gregory, *Height, Health and History: Nutritional Status in the United Kingdom* (Cambridge: Cambridge University Press, 1990), 207, 275 and 326: Landers, *Death and the Metropolis*, 354; and Roy Porter, 'Cleaning up in the Great Wen: public health in eighteenth century London' in W.F. Bynum and R. Porter (eds), *Living and Dying in London: Medical History Supplement* no. 11 (London: Wellcome Institute for the History of Medicine, 1991), 61–75. See also D. Sunderland, 'A monument to defective administration? The London Commission of Sewers in the early nineteenth century', *Urban History*, 26 (1999), 349–72.

6. Floud, Wachter and Gregory, *Height, Health and History*, 205–7, 288–95 and Simon Szreter and Graham Mooney, 'Urbanization, mortality, and the standard of living debate: new estimates of the expectation of life at birth in nineteenth century British cities', *Economic History Review*, lx (1998), 108, 110.

7. *Annual* and *Decennial Reports of the Registrar-General. Annual Report of the Medical Officer of Health: Hackney 1895*, 49–54.

8. London Metropolitan Archive. 15.0 (1899) 'London Government Bill, 1899. Report by the Medical Officer upon the Provisions of the London Government Bill', 3.

9. *Annual Report of the Medical Officer to the London County Council: 1893*, Appendix 4, 1–2: ibid., 1895, 73.

10. *Annual Report of the Medical Officer of Health to the London County Council: 1899*, Appendix 2, 1–23.

11. *Annual Report of the Medical Officer to the London County Council: 1896*, Appendix 7, 1–6.

12. M. Durey, *The Return of the Plague: British Society and the Cholera 1831–2* (Dublin: Gill and Macmillan, 1979), 50–76: S.E. Finer, *The Life and Times of Sir Edwin Chadwick* (London: Methuen, 1952), 333–54; R.A. Lewis, *Edwin Chadwick and the Public Health Movement 1832–1854* (London: Longmans, Green, 1952), ch. 9; R.S. Lambert, *Sir John Simon 1816–1904 and English Social Administration* (London: MacGibbon and Kee, 1963), 123–31 and 202–8.

13. British Parliamentary Papers (BPP) 1866, vol. xxxvii, 'Report on the Cholera Epidemic of 1866 in England', 120.

14. BPP, 1867, vol. xxxvii, 'Ninth Report of the Medical Officer of the Privy Council'.

15. See Table 3.2, 49 above.

16. BBP 1893–4, vol. xl (ii), Appendix G.1, *Report of the Royal Commission on the Water Supply of the Metropolis*, Table 11.

17. W.E. Buck, 'On infantile diarrhoea', *Transactions of the Sanitary Institute of Great Britain*, vii (1885–6), 87.

18. Naomi Williams and Graham Mooney, 'Infant mortality in an "age of great cities": London and the provincial cities, c. 1840–1914', *Continuity and Change*, 9 (1994), 191–2, Tables 1 and 2.

19. Szreter and Mooney, 'Urbanization and mortality', 88, Table 1.
20. Andrew Lees, *Cities Perceived: Urban Society in European and American Thought 1820–1940* (Manchester: Manchester University Press, 1985), 106–17.
21. E. Hart, 'Mortality statistics of healthy and unhealthy districts of London', *Sanitary Record*, vi (1879), 57.
22. Gareth Stedman Jones, *Outcast London: A Study in the Relationship between the Classes in Victorian Society* (Oxford: Oxford University Press, 1971): Daniel Pick, *Faces of Degenerationism: A European Disorder c. 1848–1914* (Cambridge: Cambridge University Press, 1989): Jose Harris, *Private Lives, Public Spirit: Britain 1870–1914* (Oxford: Oxford University Press, 1993), 241–5; and Lees, *Cities Perceived*, 136–43.
23. Owen, *Government of Victorian London*, ch. 6.
24. The best account is still A.K. Mudhopadhyay, 'The politics of London water supply, 1871–1971', Ph.D. thesis, University of London, 1972. But see also Anne Hardy, 'Water and the search for public health in London in the eighteenth and nineteenth centuries', *Medical History*, 28 (1984), 250–84 and the same author's 'Parish pump to private pipes; London's water supply in the nineteenth century' in Bynum and Porter, *Living and Dying*, 76–94. The larger national context is well described by J.A. Hassan, *A History of Water in Modern England and Wales* (Manchester: Manchester University Press, 1998).
25. Bill Luckin, *Pollution and Control: A Social History of the Thames in the Nineteenth Century* (Bristol and Boston: Adam Hilger, 1986), 81–95.
26. See, for example, BPP, 1867, vol. xxxviii, *Ninth Report of the Medical Officer of the Privy Council*, appendix 7, 'Mr J. Netten Radcliffe on cholera in London especially in the eastern districts', and BPP, 1870, vol. xxxviii, *Twelfth Annual Report of the Medical Officer of the Privy Council*, Appendix 5. 'Report by Mr J. Netten Radcliffe on the turbidity of the water supplied by certain London water companies', appendix 5.
27. See Table 3.1 above.
28. Hamlin, *Science of Impurity*.
29. Owen, *Government of Victorian London*, 133–40; Davis, *Reforming London*, 47–50; and Mudhopadhyay, 'Politics of London water supply'.
30. G.M. Ayers, *England's First State Hospitals and the Metropolitan Asylums Board, 1867–1930* (London: Wellcome Institute for the History of Medicine, 1971).
31. Graham Mooney, Bill Luckin and Andrea Tanner, 'Patient pathways: solving the problem of institutional mortality in the later nineteenth century', *Social History of Medicine*, 12 (1999), 237, Figure 1.
32. J.M. Eyler, *Victorian Social Medicine: The Ideas and Methods of William Farr* (Baltimore: Johns Hopkins University Press, 1979): M.J. Cullen, *The Statistical Movement in Early Victorian Britain* (Hassocks: Harvester Press, 1979) and 'The General Registry Office of England and Wales and the public health movement

1837–1914, a comparative perspective', *Social History of Medicine*, 4 (1991). Special issue.

33. A.S. Wohl, 'Unfit for human habitation' in H.J. Dyos and M. Wolff (eds), *The Victorian City: Images and Realities: Volume I* (London: Routledge and Kegan Paul, 1971), 610. See also Anne Hardy, 'Public health and the expert: the London medical officers of health, 1856–1900' in R.M. MacLeod (ed.), *Government and Expertise: Specialists, Administrators and Professionals, 1860–1919* (Cambridge: Cambridge University Press, 1988), 128–42.

34. On this issue, see R.M. MacLeod, 'The X-Club: A social network of science in late Victorian England', *Royal Society: Notes and Records*, 5 (1970–1), 63–72 and Adrian Desmond, *Huxley: Devil's Disciple to Evolution's High Priest* (London: Penguin Books, 1997), 327–30.

35. Useful details are contained in C.F. Brockington, 'Public health at the Privy Council 1851–71', *Medical Officer*, xci (1959), 173–7: see also the relevant biographical details in Lambert, *Sir John Simon and English Social Administration*.

36. H. Jephson, *The Sanitary Evolution of London* (London: F. Fisher Unwin, 1907), 82.

37. Ibid., 382.

38. W.A. Robson, *The Government and Misgovernment of London* (London: Allen and Unwin, 1939), 83.

39. I.G. Gibbon and R.W. Bell, *History of the London County Council 1889–1939* (London: Macmillan, 1939), 25, 27.

40. Jephson, *Sanitary Evolution*, 302, 398.

41. Sir U. Kay-Shuttleworth, *Reform of London Government: Speech in the House of Commons, 5 April 1878* (London: Municipal Reform League, 1879), 5.

42. Ibid., 18.

43. This may be concluded from Owen, *Government of Victorian London* and more emphatically from A. Clinton and P. Murray, 'Reassessing the vestries: London local government, 1855–1900' in A. O'Day (ed.), *Government and Institutions in the Post-1832 United Kingdom* (Lewiston: Edwin Mellon Press, 1995), 51–84. Davis, *London Government Problem*, ch. 1 and Dennis, 'Modern London', 101–2 are more circumspect, while Young and Garside, *Metropolitan London* p. 21, restrict themselves to the generalization that the 'vestries ... varied widely in their size, wealth and responsiveness'. (21) In *London 1808–1870: The Infernal Wen* (London: Secker and Warburg, 1971), Francis Sheppard bases his assessment of the vestries almost wholly on Jephson, *Sanitary Evolution*, a work in which these bodies are lampooned as opponents of every initiative for social and environmental reform. The same author's *London: A History* (Oxford: Oxford University Press, 1998), 284, presents a slightly more favourable view. For a balanced account of the post-revisionist consensus see S. Inwood, *A History of London* (London: Macmillan, 1998).

44. John Langton, 'Urban growth and economic change: from the late seventeenth century to 1841', in Clark, *Cambridge Urban History: Volume 2*, 473, Table 14.4 and P. Sharpe, 'Population and society 1700–1840' in the same volume at p. 500.

45. H.J. Dyos and D.A. Reeder, 'Slums and suburbs' in Dyos and Wolff, *Victorian City: Volume 1*, 359–86.

46. Luckin, *Pollution and Control*, 17–20. See, also, Stephen Halliday, *The Great Stink of London: Sir Joseph Bazalgette and the Cleansing of the Victorian Metropolis* (Stroud: Sutton, 1998). In addition to Owen, *Government of Victorian London*, explicitly or implicitly revisionist accounts of the MBW are to be found in Gloria Clifton, *Professionalism, Patronage and Public Service in Victorian London* (London: UCL Press, 1992), and D.H. Porter, *The Thames Embankment: Technology and Society in Victorian London* (Akron, OH.: University of Akron Press, 1999). For orientation on a generalized nineteenth-century provincial ethos see Briggs, *Victorian Cities*; Donald Read, *The English Provinces c.1760– 1960: A Study in Influence* (London: Edward Arnold, 1964); H.J. Dyos, 'Great and Greater London: notes on metropolis and provinces in the nineteenth and twentieth centuries', in David Cannadine and David Reeder (eds), *Exploring the Urban Past: Essays in Urban History by H.J. Dyos* (Cambridge: Cambridge University Press, 1982), 37–55: E.P. Hennock, *Fit and Proper Persons: Ideal and Reality in Nineteenth Century Urban Government* (London: Edward Arnold, 1973): L.H. Lees, 'Urban networks' in Daunton, *Cambridge Urban History: Vol.3*, 81–6: and R.J. Morris and R.H. Trainor (eds), *Urban Governance: Britain and Beyond since 1750* (Aldershot: Ashgate, 2000). See, in particular, in this volume, R.H. Trainor, 'The "decline" of British urban governance since 1750: a reassessment', 28–46.

47. Norman Davies, *The Isles: A History* (London: Macmillan, 1999), ch. 9.

48. For background here see P.J. Corfield, *The Impact of British Towns 1700–1800* (Oxford: Oxford University Press, 1982), 79–81: Bryan Keith-Lucas, *The Unreformed Government System* (London: Croom Helm, 1980); Derek Fraser, *Urban Politics in Victorian England: The Structure of Politics in Victorian Cities* (Leicester: University of Leicester Press, 1976), 55–90 and 154–77: and E.P. Hennock, 'Urban sanitary reform a generation before Chadwick?', *Economic History Review*, x (1957), 113–20. See, also, Sunderland, 'A monument to defective administration?'. Links between predominantly eighteenth and nineteenth century ways of perceiving and intervening in the urban environment are definitively described in Christopher Hamlin, *Public Health and Social Justice in the Age of Chadwick: Britain 1800–1854* (Cambridge: Cambridge University Press, 1998). Continuing conflicts between new and longer established forms of local government in provincial Britain in the period after 1835 are confronted in Derek Fraser, *Power and Authority in the Victorian City* (Oxford: Blackwell, 1979).

49. Nicholas Goddard, '"A mine of wealth": the Victorians and the agricultural value of sewage', *Journal of Historical Geography*, 22 (1996), 274–90 and John Sheail, 'Town wastes, agricultural sustainability and Victorian sewage', *Urban History*, 23 (1996), 189–210.

50. Simon Szreter, 'Economic growth, disruption, deprivation, disease and death: on the importance of the politics of public health for development', *Population*

and Development Review, 23 (1997), 698–723. See, also, Simon Szreter and Anne Hardy, 'Urban fertility and mortality patterns', in Daunton, *Cambridge Urban History*, 633–49 and J.G. Williamson, *Coping with City Growth during the British Industrial Revolution* (Cambridge: Cambridge University Press, 1990). A.S. Wohl, *Endangered Lives: Public Health in Victorian Britain* (London: Dent, 1983), 112–16, provides a succinct account of the increasing uptake of central governmental loans for public works from the 1870s onwards among increasingly politically stable municipalities.

51. Szreter and Mooney, 'Urbanization and mortality', 90, Table 2. Other work that has made use of spatial analysis and differential cause-specific death rates to examine intra-urban differentials includes M.E. Pooley and C.G. Pooley, 'Health, society and environment in nineteenth century Manchester', in Woods and Woodward, *Urban Disease and Mortality*, 148–75 and R.I. Woods, 'Mortality and sanitary conditions in the 'best governed city in the world', *Journal of Historical Geography*, 4 (1978), 35–56.

52. 'London health in 1908', *Sanitary Record*, xliv (1909), 623.

53. An exception is Anne Hardy, *The Epidemic Streets: Infectious Disease and the Rise of Preventive Medicine 1856–1900* (Oxford: Clarendon Press, 1993). Emphatically non-political in the conventional sense of the term, this study nevertheless reveals a great deal about bureaucratic conflict and compromise at local level. In *The Government of Victorian London*, John Owen confirms that in the capital, as in urban provincial Britain, differences over public health policies could trigger open political warfare. See, in particular, the Southwark fever saga of the 1860s, involving the irrepressible one-time medical officer and vestryman George Rendle, 306–312.

54. Cited in Waller, *Town, City and Nation*, 63.

55. *Report of the County Council to 31st. March, 1919* (London: London County Council, 1920), 11.

56. Ibid., 9, 11, 15.

57. See Andrew Saint (ed.), *Politics and the People of London: The London County Council 1889–1965* (London: Hambledon, 1989) and S.D. Pennybacker, *A Vision for London: London, Everyday Life and the LCC Experiment* (London: Routledge, 1995).

58. Richard Dennis begins to explore this terrain in 'Modern London'.

Chapter 6   Pollution in the City

1. The best existing study is A.S. Wohl, *Endangered Lives: Public Health in Victorian Britain* (London: Dent, 1983). But see also Keith Thomas, *Man and the Natural World: Changing Attitudes in England 1500–1800* (London: Weidenfeld and Nicolson, 1983): P. Brimblecombe and C. Pfister (eds), *Silent Countdown: Essays in European Environmental History* (London and Berlin: Springer-Verlag, 1990): and Michael Shortland (ed.), *Science and Nature: Essays in the History of the*

Environmental Sciences (Stamford in the Vale: British Society for the History of Science, 1993). In addition, the writings of Christopher Hamlin, liberally cited below, are seminal. J A. Hassan, *Prospects for Economic and Environmental History* (Manchester: Department of Economic History, Manchester Metropolitan University, 1995) outlines the larger historiographical situation.

2. For North America see Martin V. Melosi (ed.), *Pollution and Reform in American Cities 1870–1930* (Austin, TX: University of Texas Press, 1980): K.E. Bailes, *Environmental History: Critical Issues in Comparative Perspective* (Lanham: University Press of America, 1985): and Joel A. Tarr, *The Search for the Ultimate Sink: Urban Pollution in Historical Perspective* (Akron, Ohio: University of Akron Press, 1996). On France see A. Corbin, *The Foul and the Fragrant: Odour and the French Social Imaignation* (Leamington Spa: Berg, 1986), translated by M.L. Kochan; D. Reid, *Paris Sewers and Sewermen: Realities and Representations* (Cambridge, Mass.: Harvard University Press, 1991); and A.F. Laberge, *Mission and Method: The Early Nineteenth Century French Public Health Movement* (Cambridge: Cambridge University Press, 1992).

3. Mary Douglas, *Purity and Danger: An Analysis of Concepts of Pollution and Taboo* (London: Routledge, 1966): Mary Douglas, 'Environments at risk', in Douglas, *Implicit Meanings: Selected Essays in Anthropology* (London: Routledge, 1999), 230–48; and Mary Doulgas and Aaron Wildavsky, *Risk and Culture: An Essay on the Selection of Technical and Environmental Dangers* (Berkeley and London: University of California Press, 1982). See also Ulrich Beck, *The Risk Society: Towards a New Modernity* (London: Sage, 1992). Translated by M. Ritter and Brian Wynne, *Rationality and Ritual: The Windscale Inquiry and Nuclear Decisions in Britain* (Chalfont St Giles: British Society for the History of Science, 1982).

4. Douglas, 'Environments at risk'; Douglas and Wildavsky, *Risk and Culture* and Christopher Hamlin, 'Environmental sensibility in Edinburgh, 1839–1840: the fetid irrigation controversy', *Journal of Urban History,* 20 (1994), 311–39.

5. G. Rosen, 'Disease, debility and death', in H.J. Dyos and M. Wolff (eds), *The Victorian City: Volume Two* (London: Routledge and Kegan Paul, 1973), 650-I. See also P. Townsend, N. Davidson and M. Whitehead (eds), *Inequalities in Health: The Black Report* (Harmondsworth: Penguin Books, 1988), 43–5, 228–9 and 274–6.

6. Naomi Williams, 'Death in its season: class, environment and the mortality of infants in nineteenth-century Sheffield', *Social History of Medicine,* 5 (1992), 71–94; Naomi Williams and Graham Mooney, 'Infant mortality in an "age of great cities": London and the English provincial cities compared, *c.*1840–1910', *Continuity and Change,* 9 (1994), 185–212; and Barbara Thompson, 'Infant mortality in nineteenth-century Bradford', in Robert Woods and John Woodward (eds), *Urban Disease and Mortality in Nineteenth-Century England* (London: Batsford, 1984), 120–47.

7. C. H. Lee, 'Regional inequalities in infant mortality in Britain, 1871–1971: patterns and hypotheses', *Population Studies,* 45 (1991), 55–65; and E. Garrett and A. Reid, '"Satanic mills, pleasant lands": spatial variation in women's work

and infant mortality as viewed from the 1911 *Census*', *Historical Research,* 68 (1994), 156–77.

8. T. C. Barker and J. R. Harris, *A Merseyside Town in the Industrial Revolution: St Helens 1750–1900* (Liverpool: University of Liverpool Press, 1954); A. E. Dingle, '"The monster nuisance of all": landowners, alkali manufacturers and air pollution 1828–1864', *Economic History Review,* 35 (1982), 529–48; and R. Rees, 'The South Wales copper-smoke dispute, 1828–95', *Welsh History Review,* 10 (1981), 480–96.

9. E. Le Roy Ladurie, 'A concept: the unification of the globe by disease (fourteenth to sixteenth centuries)', in Ladurie, *The Mind and Method of the Historian* (Chicago: University of Chicago Press, 1981), 28–83. Translated by S. and B. Reynolds. See also A. W. Crosby, *Ecological Imperialism: The Biological Expansion of Europe 900–1900* (Cambridge: Cambridge University Press, 1986), ch. 9.

10. Lawrence Stone, *The Crisis of the Aristocracy* (Oxford: Oxford University Press, 1965), 386–96: Raymond Williams, *The Country and the City* (London: Hogarth Press, 1973); P. J. Corfield, *The Impact of English Towns 1700–1800* (Oxford: Oxford University Press, 1982), ch. 5; and Thomas, *Man and the Natural World,* 243–54. For a comparative perspective see the path-breaking William Cronon, *Nature's Metropolis: Chicago and the Great West* (New York: Norton, 1991), ch. 8.

11. R. M. Macleod, 'Government and resource conservation: the Salmon Acts Administration, 1860–1886', *Journal of British Studies,* 8 (1968), 114–50. See also Peter Bartrip, 'Food for the body and food for the mind: the regulation of freshwater fisheries in the 1870s', *Victorian Studies,* 28 (1985), 285–304.

12. R. M. MacLeod, 'The Alkali Acts administration, 1863–84: the emergence of the civil scientist', *Victorian Studies,* 9 (1965), 85–112.

13. H. Heimann, 'Effects of air pollution on human health', in *Air Pollution* (Geneva: World Health Organisation, Monograph 46, 1961), 172–6; and W. P. D. Logan, 'Mortality in the London fog accident, 1952', *The Lancet,* i (1953), 336–8.

14. R. Hawes, 'The municipal regulation of smoke pollution in Liverpool, 1853–1866', *Environment and History,* 4 (1998), 75–90. See also C. Bowler and P. Brimblecombe, 'The difficulties of abating smoke in late Victorian York', *Atmospheric Environment,* 24B (1990), 49–55.

15. E. Ashby and M. Anderson, *The Politics of Clean Air* (Oxford: Oxford University Press, 1981), 16–17.

16. A. Elliot, 'Municipal government in Bradford in the mid-nineteenth century', in Derek Fraser (ed.), *Municipal Reform and the Industrial City* (Leicester: Leicester University Press, 1982), 123–4.

17. B. Barber, 'Municipal government in Leeds, 1835–1914', in Fraser, *Municipal Reform,* 75–6.

18. Carlos Flick, 'The movement for smoke abatement in nineteenth-century Britain', *Technology and Culture,* 21 (1980), 50.

19. Christopher Hamlin, 'Providence and putrefaction: Victorian sanitarians and the natural theology of health and disease', *Victorian Studies,* 28 (1984–5), 393. See also J. F. Brenner, 'Nuisance law and the industrial revolution', *Journal of Legal Studies,* 3 (1974), 403–33.

20. T. F. Glick, 'Science, technology and the urban environment: the Great Stink of 1858' in L. J. Bilsky (ed.), *Historical Ecology* (Port Washington: Kennikat Press, 1980), 122–39; and Bill Luckin, *Pollution and Control: A Social History of the Thames in the Nineteenth Century* (Bristol and Boston: Adam Hilger, 1986), 17–20.

21. Douglas, *Purity and Danger*; Christopher Hamlin, 'Edward Frankland's career as London's official water analyst 1865–1876: the context of "previous sewage contamination"', *Bulletin of the History of Medicine,* 56 (1982), 56–76; Hamlin, 'Providence and putrefaction'; and R. L. Schoenwald, 'Training urban man', in Dyos and Wolff, *Victorian City, Vol. 2,* 669–92.

22. R. A. Lewis, *Edwin Chadwick and the Public Health Movement 1832–1854* (London: Longmans, Green, 1952), ch. 2; Christopher Hamlin, 'Edwin Chadwick and the engineers, 1842–1854: systems and anti-systems in the pipe-and-brick sewers war', *Technology and Culture,* 33 (1992), 680–709; and Graeme Davison, 'The city as a natural system: theories of urban society in early nineteenth-century Britain', in Derek Fraser and Anthony Sutcliffe (eds), *The Pursuit of Urban History* (London: Edward Arnold, 1983), 349–70.

23. Wohl, *Endangered Lives,* 95. See also M. J. Daunton, *House and Home in the Victorian City* (London: Edward Arnold, 1983), 248.

24. A. Redford and I. S. Russell, *The History of Local Government in Manchester: Volume 111: The Last Half Century* (London: Longmans, 1940), 128. See also A. Wilson, 'Technology and municipal decision-making: sanitary systems in Manchester, 1868–1910', Ph.D. thesis, University of Manchester, 1990.

25. O. Checkland and M. Lamb (eds), *Health Care as Social History: The Glasgow Case* (Aberdeen: University of Aberdeen Press, 1982), 6; and R. A. Cage, 'Health in Glasgow' in Cage (ed.), *The Working-Class in Glasgow* (London: Croom Helm), 68.

26. P. J. Smith, 'The foul burns of Edinburgh: public health attitudes and environmental change', *Scottish Geographical Magazine,* 91 (1975), 25–37 and Smith, 'The legislated control over river pollution in Victorian Scotland', *Scottish Geographical Magazine,* 98 (1982), 66–76. See also Hamlin, 'Environmental sensibility'.

27. I. Budge and C. O'Leary, *Belfast: Approach to Crisis: A Study of Belfast Politics 1613–1970* (London: Macmillan, 1973), 110–11. On similar conditions in urban Ireland see J. V. O'Brien, *'Dear Dirty Dublin': A City in Distress 1899–1916* (Berkeley: University of California Press, 1982), 18–19.

28. G. Roberts, *Aspects of Welsh History* (Cardiff: University of Wales Press, 1969), 145–55.

29. Barber, 'Municipal government', 67–70; and B. J. Barber, 'Aspects of municipal government, 1835–1914' in D. Fraser (ed.), *A History of Modern Leeds* (Manchester: Manchester University Press, 1980), 301–26.

30. W. E. Bijker, T. P. Hughes and T. J. Pinch (eds), *The Social Construction of Technological Systems: New Directions in the Sociology and History of Technology* (Cambridge, Mass.: MIT Press, 1992): W.E. Bijker and John Law (eds), *Shaping Technology/ Building Society: Studies in Sociotechnical Change* (Cambridge: Mass., MIT Press, 1992) and Langdon Winner, 'Upon opening the black box and finding it empty: social constructivism and the philosophy of technology', *Science, Technology and Human Values,* 18 (1993), 362–78.

31. Christopher Hamlin, 'Muddling in bumbledom: on the enormity of large sanitary improvements in four British towns, 1855–1885', *Victorian Studies,* 33 (1988–9), 55–83.

32. Nicholas Goddard, '"A mine of wealth": the Victorians and the agricultural value of sewage', *Journal of Historical Geography,* 22 (1996), 274–90; and John Sheail, 'Town wastes, agricultural sustainability and Victorian sewage', *Urban History,* 23 (1996) 189–210.

33. British Parliamentary Papers (BPP) 1870, vol. xi, *Second Report of the Rivers Pollution Commissioners: The A.B.C. Process of Treating Sewage,* 449 *passim.*

34. F. E. Bruce, 'Water supply and waste disposal', in T. I. Williams (ed.), *A History of Technology, Volume Seven: The Twentieth Century c. 1890 to c. 1950* (Oxford: Oxford University Press, 1958), 1382–98. See also Christopher Hamlin, 'William Dibdin and the idea of biological sewage treatment', *Technology and Culture,* 29 (1988), 189–218.

35. Ministry of Housing and Local Government, *Taken for Granted: Report of the Working Party on Sewage Disposal* (London: HMSO, 1970), 7.

36. H. S. Tinker, 'The problem', in Institution of Civil Engineers, *Advances in Sewage Treatment* (London: Institute of Civil Engineers, 1973), 3–4. See also John Sheail, 'Sewering the English suburbs: an inter-war perspective', *Journal of Historical Geography,* 19 (1993), 433–47 and Sheail, 'Taken for granted": the inter-war West Middlesex Drainage Scheme', *London Journal,* 18 (1993), 143–56.

37. Tinker, 'Problem', 5.

38. L. B. Wood, *The Restoration of the Tidal Thames* (Bristol: Adam Hilger, 1982).

39. B. W. Clapp, *An Environmental History of Britain since the Industrial Revolution* (London: Routledge, 1994), 89.

40. John Sheail, 'Public interest and self-interest: the disposal of trade effluent in inter-war Britain', *Twentieth Century British History,* 4 (1993), 149–70.

41. Clapp, *Environmental History,* 89.

42. A. Wheeler, *The Tidal Thames* (London: Routledge and Kegan Paul, 1979), ch. 4.

43. J. A. Hassan, 'The water industry, 1900–1951: a failure of public policy?' in R. Millward and J. Singleton (eds), *The Political Economy of Nationalisation, 1920–1950* (Cambridge: Cambridge University Press, 1995), 189–211.

44. J. A. Hassan, *Environmental and Economic History,* 9.

45. M. Sigsworth and M. Worboys, 'The public's view of public health in mid-Victorian Britain', *Urban History*, 21 (1994), 243–4.

46. J. A. Hassan, 'The growth and impact of the British water industry in the nineteenth century', *Economic History Review*, 38 (1985), 531–47.

47. Wohl, *Endangered Lives*, 62.

48. I. H. Adams, *The Making of Urban Scotland* (London: Croom Helm, 1978), 136.

49. R. K. J. Grant, 'Merthyr Tydfil in the mid-nineteenth century: the struggle for public health', *Welsh History Review*, 14 (1989), 574–94. See also Geoffrey Best, *Mid-Victorian Britain 1851–75* (London: Fontana, 1971), 45–6.

50. See Anne Hardy, 'Urban famine or urban crisis? Typhus in the Victorian city', *Medical History*, 32 (1988), 419 n. 133: Hardy, 'Water and the search for public health in London in the eighteenth and nineteenth centuries', *Medical History*, 28 (1984), 250–84 and Hardy, 'Parish pump to private pipes: London's water supply in the nineteenth century', in W. F. Bynum and R. Porter (eds), *Living and Dying in London* (London: Wellcome Institute for the History of Medicine, *Medical History Supplement* no. 11, 1991), 76–93.

51. N. M. Blake, *Water for the Cities: A History of the Urban Water Supply Problem in the United States* (New York: University of Syracuse Press, 1956), 264.

52. John Stevenson, *British Society 1914–45* (Harmondsworth: Penguin Books, 1984), 210.

53. P. J. Waller, *Town, City and Nation* (Oxford: Oxford University Press, 1983), 301–2.

54. F. McKichan, 'A burgh's response to the problems of urban growth: Stirling, 1780–1880', *Scottish Historical Review*, 57 (1978), 68–86. See also G. Kearns, 'Cholera, nuisances and environmental management in Islington, 1830–1855' in Bynum and Porter, *Living and Dying*, 76–93.

55. Anne Hardy, *The Epidemic Streets: Infectious Disease and the Rise of Preventive Medicine 1856–1900* (Oxford: Clarendon Press, 1993), 189 n. 173.

56. F. Flintoff and R. Millard, *Public Cleansing* (London: Maclaren, 1969), 1–2. See also W. A. Robson, *The Government and Misgovernment of London* (London; Allen and Unwin, 1939), 201–12.

57. M. Gandy, *Recycling and the Politics of Urban Waste* (London: Earthscan, 1994), 42. See also the same author's *Waste and Recycling* (Aldershot: Avebury, 1993).

58. Asa Briggs, *Victorians Things* (Stroud: Sutton, 1988), 27.

59. Gandy, *Waste and Recycling*, 42.

60. Ibid., 40.

61. Department of the Environment, *Refuse Disposal: Report of the Working Party on Refuse Disposal* (London: HMSO, 1971), 8–9.

62. Mark Jenner, 'The politics of London air: John Evelyn's *Fumifugium* and the Restoration', *Historical Journal*, 38 (1995), 535–51.

63. Clapp, *Environmental History*, 43.

64. BPP 1844, vol. xvii, *First Report of the Commissioners for Inquiring into the State of Large Towns and Populous Districts*, 43.

65. Neil Arnott, 'On a new smoke consuming and fuel-saving fire place', *Journal of the Society of Arts,* 1–2 (1852–4), 428–35. Comment by Edwin Chadwick, 435.

66. MacLeod, 'Alkali acts'.

67. Ibid., 86.

68. 'Advantages of the fog', *The Lancet,* i (1892), 1433; and H. C. Bartlett, 'Some of the present aspects of practical sanitation', *Transactions of the Sanitary Institute of Great Britain,* 6 (1844–5), 44–5.

69. Anne Hardy, 'Rickets and the rest: childcare, diet and the infectious children's diseases', *Social History of Medicine,* 5 (1992), 389–412.

70. The literature on this theme is now large but a comprehensive bibliography is contained in Daniel Pick, *Faces of Degeneration: A European Disorder c. 1848– 1918* (Cambridge, 1989). See also the classic formulations in Gareth Stedman Jones, *Outcast London: A Study of the Relationship between Classes in Victorian Society* (Oxford: Oxford University Press, 1971), 127–9, 149–51 and 286–7.

71. W. S. Jevons, *The Coal Question: An Enquiry Concerning the Progress of the Nation* (Basingstoke: Palgrave, 2001), reprint edition; P. Brantlinger (ed.), *Energy and Entropy: Science and Culture in Nineteenth Century Britain: Essays from Victorian Studies* (Bloomington: Indian University Press, 1989) and Briggs, *Victorian Things,* 298–308.

72. Stephen Mosely, 'The Manchester and Salford Noxious Vapour Abatement Association, 1876–1895', M.A. thesis, Lancaster University, 1994.

73. J. B. Cohen, 'A record of the work of the Leeds Smoke Abatement Society', *Journal of the Royal Sanitary Institute,* 27 (1906), 71–3. For a revealing North American comparison see H. L. Platt, 'Invisible gases: smoke, gender and the redefinition of environmental policy in Chicago, 1900–1920', *Planning Perspectives,* 10 (1995), 67–97.

74. H. T. Bernstein, 'The mysterious disappearance of Edwardian London fog', *London Journal,* 2 (1975), 189–206.

75. W. A. L. Marshall, *A Century of London Weather* (London: HMSO, 1952), 42–53; J. H. Brazell, *London Weather* (London: HMSO, 1968): and T. J. Chandler, *The Climate of London* (London: Hutchinson, 1965), ch. 12.

76. On Manchester, in particular, see J. B. Priestley, *English Journey* (Harmonds-worth: Penguin Books, 1987), 237–48. On twentieth century pressure group activity see E. Ashby and M. Anderson, 'Studies in the politics of environmental protection: the historical roots of the British Clean Air Act, 1956. II. The ripening of public opinion, 1898–1952', *Interdisciplinary Science Reviews,* 2 (1977), 190–206. Issues of representation and reform during this period are confronted by Tim Boon in 'The smoke menace: cinema, sponsorship and the social relations of science in 1937' in Shortland, *Science and Nature,* 57–87.

77. Heimann, 'Effects of air pollution' and Logan, 'Mortality'.

78. E. H. Blake and W. R. Jenkins, *Drainage and Sanitation* (London: Batsford, 1956), 479.

79. J. G. Williamson, 'Did England's cities grow too fast during the Industrial Revolution?' in P. Higonnet, D. S. Landes and H. Rosovsky (eds), *Favorites of*

Fortune: Technology, Growth and Economic Development since the Industrial Revolution (Cambridge, Mass.: Harvard University Press, 1991), 390–1. See also J. G. Williamson, *Coping with City Growth during the British Industrial Revolution* (Cambridge: Cambridge University Press, 1990), and particularly chs. 8–10.

Chapter 7   'The Heart and Home of Horror': The Great London Fogs of the Late Nineteenth Century

1. See in particular Roy Porter and Dorothy Porter, *In Sickness and In Health: The British Experience* (Oxford: Polity Press,1988): Roy Porter, 'Laymen, doctors and medical knowledge in the eighteenth century: the evidence of the *Gentleman's Magazine*' in Porter (ed.), *Patients and Practitioners: Lay Perceptions of Medicine in Pre-Industrial Society* (Cambridge: Cambridge University Press, 1985), 281– 314 and Porter, *Mind-Forg'd Manacles: Madness and Psychiatry in England from the Restoration to the Regency* (Cambridge: Mass.: Harvard University Press, 1985).

2. A.S. Wohl, *Endangered Lives: Public Health in Victorian Britain* (London: Dent, 1983): Anne Hardy, *The Epidemic Streets: Infectious Disease and the Rise of Preventive Medicine 1856–1900* (Oxford: Clarendon Press, 1993): Nancy Tomes, *The Gospel of Germs: Men, Women and the Microbe in American Life* (Cambridge, Mass.: Harvard University Press,1998) and Michael Worboys, *Spreading Germs: Disease Theories and Medical Practice in Britain 1865–1900* (Cambridge: Cambridge University Press, 2000).

3. Christopher Hamlin, *A Science of Impurity: Water Analysis in Nineteenth Century Britain* (Berkeley: University of California Press, 1990) and *Public Health and Social Justice in the Age of Chadwick: Britain 1800–54* (Cambridge: Cambridge University Press, 1998).

4. Thomas McKeown, *The Modern Rise of Population* (London: Edward Arnold, 1976). For an overview of the current consensus see Simon Szreter and Anne Hardy, 'Urban fertility and mortality patterns' in Martin Daunton (ed.), *The Cambridge Urban History of Britain: Volume 3: 1750–1840* (Cambridge: Cambridge University Press, 2000), 629–73. Robert Woods and Nicola Shelton, *An Atlas of Victorian Mortality* (Liverpool: Liverpool University Press, 1997) and Robert I. Woods, *The Demography of Victorian England and Wales* (Cambridge University Press, 2000) pinpoint major technical and interpretative innovation.

5. Joel A.Tarr, *The Search for the Ultimate Sink: Urban Pollution in Historical Perspective* (Akron, OH. University of Akron Press, 1995); William Cronon, *Nature's Metropolis: Chicago and the Great West* (New York: Norton, 1991); and Martin V. Melosi, *Effluent America: Cities, Industry, Energy and the Environment* (Pittsburgh: University of Pittsburgh Press, 2001). The 'anti-urban' position has been authoritatively articulated by Donald Worster, 'Transformations of the earth: toward an agroecological perspective in history', *Journal of American*

History, 77 (1990), 1087–106. For recent and distinctive European developments see P. Brimblecombe and C. Pfister (eds), *Silent Countdown: Essays in European Environmental History* (London and Berlin: Springer-Verlag, 1990) and Christoph Bernhardt and Genevieve Massard-Guilbaud (eds), *The Modern Demon: Pollution in Urban and Industrial European Societies* (Clermont-Ferrand: Presses Universitaires Blaise-Pascal, 2002).

6. B.W.Clapp, *An Environmental History of Britain since the Industrial Revolution* (London: Longman, 1994) and John Sheail, *An Environmental History of Twentieth Century Britain* (Basingstoke: Palgrave, 2002). But see also Wohl, *Endangered Lives*, 205–56.

7. Stephen Mosley, *The Chimney of the World: A History of Smoke Pollution in Victorian and Edwardian Manchester* (Cambridge: White Horse Press, 2001). See, for a comprehensive transatlantic overview, David Stradling, *Smokestacks and Progressives: Environmentalists, Engineers, and Air Quality 1881–1951* (Baltimore: Johns Hopkins University Press, 1999) and, for a rare venture into comparative environmental history, David Stradling and Peter Thorsheim, 'The smoke of great cities: British and American efforts to control air pollution', *Environmental History*, 4 (1999), 6–31. For a general *longue duree* account of London see Peter Brimblecombe, *The Big Smoke: A History of Air Pollution in London since Medieval Times* (London: Methuen, 1988). For a rare analysis of community conflict over water see R.K. J. Grant, 'Merthyr Tydfil in the mid-nineteenth century: the struggle for public health', *Welsh History Review*, 14 (1989), 574–94. An overview of the development of the supply industry is provided in J.A. Hassan, *A History of Water in Modern England and Wales* (Manchester: Manchester University Press, 1998).

8. But see Christopher Hamlin, 'Environmental sensibility in Edinburgh, 1839–40: the fetid irrigation controversy', *Journal of Urban History*, 20 (1994), 311–39 and chapter 6 above. For a suggestive framework of analysis for these issues see Mary Douglas, *Purity and Danger: An Analysis of the Concepts of Pollution and Taboo* (London: Routledge and Kegan Paul, 1966); Mary Douglas, 'Environments at risk' in Douglas, *Implicit Meanings: Selected Essays in Anthropology* (London: Routledge, 1975), 230–48; and Mary Douglas and Aaron Wildavsky, *Risk and Culture: An Essay on the Selection of Technical and Environmental Dangers* (Berkeley and London: University of California Press, 1982).

9. S.E. Finer, *The Life and Times of Sir Edwin Chadwick* (London: Methuen, 1952), 333–54: R.A. Lewis, *Edwin Chadwick and the Public Health Movement 1832–1854* (London: Longman, Green, 1952), ch. 9 and 353 *passim*: and R.S. Lambert, *Sir John Simon 1816–1904 and English Social Administration* (London: MacGibbon and Kee, 1963), 123–31 and 202–8.

10. Bill Luckin, *Pollution and Control: A Social History of the Thames in the Nineteenth Century* (Bristol and Boston: Adam Hilger, 1986), 35–51.

11. *Gentleman's Magazine*, cxv (1814), 87. On the Lisbon earthquake, see E.L. Jones, *The European Miracle: Environments, Economies and Geopolitics in the History of*

Europe and Asia (Cambridge: Cambridge University Press, 1981), 26–7 and 139–40. The incidence of fog in the later eighteenth century capital is briefly documented in Clapp, *Environmental History*, 43 and R.C. Mossman, 'The non-instrumental meteorology of London, 1713–1896', *Quarterly Journal of the Royal Meteorological Society of London*, xxiii (1897), 287–98.

12. William Bent, *Remarks on the State of the Air, Vegetation etc. November, 1796* (London, 1794–1801), 25.

13. Thomas Bateman, *Reports on the Diseases of London and the State of the Weather from 1804 to 1816* (London, 1819), 185. For additional contextual information on the fog crisis of 1813–14 see *Gentleman's Magazine*, cxiv (1813), *Supplement*, 695: 'Extraordinary fog', *Annals of Philosophy*, iii (1814), 154–5 and Luke Howard, *The Climate of London: Volume 3* (London, 1833), 224.

14. *The Times*, 5 Jan. 1814.

15. Howard, *Climate of London: Vol. 2*, 207–8.

16. Howard, *Climate of London: Vol. 3*, 341.

17. J.H. Brazell, *London Weather* (London: HMSO, 1968), 102. However, there was unusually foggy weather in 1837. See *The Times*, Dec. 4 1837.

18. British Parliamentary Papers (BPP), *Select Committee on Smoke Nuisance*, 1843, vol. vii, q.2,083, evidence of A. Ure. See also *The Times*, Feb. 22 1843.

19. James Glaisher, 'On weather during the quarter ending December 31st., 1853', *Sixteenth Annual Report of the Registrar-General* (London, HMSO, 1856), cv.

20. *The Builder*, xi (1853), 613.

21. *The Globe*, Jan. 24 1865: see also *The Times*, Jan. 11 1861 and 'Fog in a metropolitan light', *The Builder*, xxiii (1865), 537–8.

22. W.P.D. Logan, 'Mortality in the London fog incident, 1952', *The Lancet*, i, (1953), 338

23. F.J. Brodie, 'On the prevalence of fog in London during the 20 years 1871 to 1890', *Quarterly Journal of the Royal Meteorological Society*, xviii (1892), 40–3 and R.H. Scott, 'Fifteen years' fogs in the British islands', *Quarterly Journal of the Royal Meteorological Society*, xix (1893), 232.

24. F.J. Brodie, 'Decrease of fog in London during recent years', *Symons Monthly Meteorological Magazine*, xxxix (1904), 213.

25. F.A.R. (Rollo) Russell, *London Fogs* (London: E. Stanford, 1880), 22–4.

26. F.A.R. (Rollo) Russell, *Smoke in Relation to Fogs in London* (London: National Smoke Abatement Office, 1889), 9.

27. Sir James Crichton-Browne, 'The dust problem', *Transactions of the Sanitary Institute of Great Britain*, xxiii (1902), 217.

28. D.J. Russell Duncan, 'On smoke abatement', *Transactions of the Sanitary Institute of Great Britain*, ix (1887–8), 317.

29. L.C.W. Bonacina, 'London fogs – then and now', *Weather*, 5 (1950), 91. See, also, the same author's 'An estimation of the Great London Fog of 5–8 December, 1952', *Weather*, 7 (1953), 333–4.

30. Bonacina, 'London fogs', 92.

31. M.W. Flinn (ed.), *Report on the Sanitary Condition of the Labouring Population of Great Britain by Edwin Chadwick 1842* (Edinburgh: Edinburgh University Press, 1965), 356–7.
32. Ibid., 273.
33. Ibid., 274.
34. B.P.P., *First Report of the Commissioners for Inquiring into the State of Large Towns and Populous Districts*, 1844, vol. xvii, 42–3.
35. Ibid., q. 251. Evidence of Thomas Cubitt.
36. William Guy, 'Effect of smoke on buildings', *The Builder*, v (1847), 498.
37. *Hansard's Parliamentary Debates (HL)*, 3rd series, vol. cxxix, Aug. 16 1853, col. 1,753.
38. Neil Arnott, 'On a new smoke-consuming and fuel saving fire-place', *Journal of the Society of Arts*, i-ii (1852–4), 428–35. Arnott's interest in these issues reached back more than 20 years. He was the author of the influential *On Warming and Ventilating* (London: Longman, 1838) and *On the Smokeless Fireplace* (London: Longman,1855).
39. W.S. Jevons, *The Coal Question: An Enquiry Concerning the Progress of the Nation* (Basingstoke: Palgrave, 2001), reprint edition. See, also, on this issue, Asa Briggs, *Victorian Things* (Stroud: Sutton, 1988), 298–308: and P. Brantlinger (ed.), *Energy and Entropy: Science and Culture in Victorian Britain: Selected Essays from Victorian Studies* (Bloomington: Indiana University Press, 1988).
40. Edwin Chadwick's spoken comments on Arnott, 'Smoke-consuming fireplace', 435.
41. F.A.R. (Rollo) Russell remains an elusive and under-documented figure. But for glimpses of his character and moral preoccupations – and oddities – see Ray Monk, *Bertrand Russell: Volume One: The Spirit of Solitude* (London: Cape, 1996), 15–19. On Russell as environmental activist and anti-fog propagandist, see E. Ashby and M. Anderson, *The Politics of Clean Air* (Oxford: Oxford University Press, 1981), 55–6.
42. F.A.R. (Rollo) Russell, *National Strategy Against Infection* (London: National Press Agency, 1888), 13.
43. Russell, *Smoke in Relation to Fogs*, 24–6.
44. *Nature*, xxxi (1884–5), 348.
45. B.P.P., *Select Committee (HL) Smoke Nuisance Abatement*, 1887, vol. xii, q. 433. Evidence of Ernest Hart. For biographical information on this important mid- and late nineteenth century public health reformer and publicist see Peter Bartrip, 'The *British Medical Journal*: a retrospect' in W.F. Bynum, R.S. Porter and Stephen Lock (eds), *Medical Journals and Medical Knowledge* (London: Routledge,1992), 126–45 and Bill Luckin, 'The shaping of a public environmental sphere in late nineteenth-century London' in S. Sturdy (ed.), *Medicine, Health and the Public Sphere* (London: Routledge, 2002), 224–40.
46. *SC Smoke Nuisance*, q. 400 *passim*, evidence of Ernest Hart.
47. 'The fog and gas consumption', *Symons Monthly Meteorological Magazine*, xxiv (Feb. 1889), 8.

48. *Hansard's Parliamentary Debates (HL)*, 4th series, vol. ix, 2 March 1891, col. 1,916.
49. 'Town fogs', *Symons Monthly Meteorological Magazine*, xxvii (Feb. 1892), 1.
50. A.Moresby White, 'The coal smoke nuisance'; *Journal of State Medicine*, ix (1901), 652.
51. M.Agar, 'The effect of smoke on plant life', *Journal of the Royal Sanitary Institute*, xxvii (1906), 175.
52. *SC Smoke Nuisance*, q. 403, evidence of Ernest Hart. On the cultural significance of the domestic grate see R.L. Patten, '"A surprising transformation": Dickens and the hearth' in C. Knopflmacher and G.B. Tennyson (eds), *Nature and the Victorian Imagination* (Berkeley: University of California, 1977), 153–70.
53. Bent, *Observations*, 5.
54. Robert Willan, *Reports on the Diseases in London* ... (London, 1801), 300.
55. Bateman, *Reports*, 134.
56. B.B.P., *Select Committee on Steam Engines and Furnaces*, 1819, vol. viii, 280–1. Evidence of George Tuthill: *SC. Smoke Nuisance*, qs, 1,927–31. Evidence of William Brande: and 'The smoke nuisance', *The Builder*, i (1843), 346.
57. 'Smoke consumption', *The Builder*, x (1852), 616 and Russell Duncan, 'On smoke abatement', 317.
58. *SC Smoke Nuisance*, q. 2,080, evidence of Andrew Ure.
59. J.A. Hingeston, 'The atmosphere in relation to disease', *Journal of Public Health and Sanitary Review*, i (1855), 354–5. See, also, *Anon*, 'Air and ventilation', *Journal of Public Health and Sanitary Review*, ii (1856), 193–220 and the comments of Dr Gibbon, medical officer of health for Holborn in 'The smoke nuisance', *The Builder*, xx (1862), 284.
60. E.Ray Lancaster, 'Fresh air', *Popular Science Review*, iii (1864), 7.
61. See, on these issues, J.W. Burrow, *Evolution and Society: A Study in Victorian Social Theory* (Cambridge: Cambridge University Press, 1966): Gay Weber, 'Science and society in nineteenth century anthropology', *History of Science*, 7 (1974), 260–83: Wohl, *Endangered Lives*, 260 and 283 and the same author's *The Eternal Slum: Housing and Social Policy in Victorian London* (London: Edward Arnold, 1977), 45–72: Gertrude Himmelfarb, *The Idea of Poverty: England in the Early Industrial Age* (New York: Knopf, 1984), 323–32; and Eileen Yeo, 'Mayhew as social investigator' in E.P. Thompson and E. Yeo (eds), *The Unknown Mayhew: Selections from the Morning Chronicle 1849–50* (Harmondsworth: Penguin, 1973), 99–100.
62. The context for this strand of thought in relation to the capital has been authoritatively established by Gareth Stedman Jones, *Outcast London: A Study in the Relationship between Classes in Victorian Society* (Oxford: Oxford University Press, 1971). See also G.E. Searle, *Eugenics and Politics in Britain 1900–1914* (Leyden: Noordoff, 1976): Greta Jones, *Social Darwinism in English Thought: The Interraction between Biological and Social Theory* (Brighton: Harvester Press, 1980): Daniel Pick, *Faces of Degeneration: A European Disorder c.1848–1918* (Cambridge: Cambridge University Press, 1989); Dorothy Porter, '"Enemies of

the race": biologism, environmentalism and public health in Edwardian Britain', *Victorian Studies*, 34 (1991), 159–78: and Jose Harris, *Private Lives, Public Spirit, Britain 1870–1914* (Oxford: Oxford University Press, 1993), 241–5.

63. See H.D. Rawnsley, 'Sunlight or smoke?', *Contemporary Review*, lvii (1891), 871 and F.A.R. (Rollo) Russell, *The Atmosphere in Relation to Human Life and Health* (Washington, D.C.: Smithsonian Miscellaneous Collections, xxxix, 1896), 90.

64. Isolation and physical disorientation attributable to metropolitan fog were well established themes. See *The Times*, Nov. 1, 1861: A.E. Fletcher, 'Pollution of the atmosphere by coal smoke', *Journal of State Medicine*, v (1900), 2: W. Mercat, 'On fogs', *Quarterly Journal of the Royal Meteorological Society*, xv (1889), 64; and Bonacina, 'London fogs', 91–3.

65. This moral journey – or purported retrogression – is elaborated in Russell, *London Fogs*, 30–2 and the same author's *Smoke in Relation to Fogs*, 21–2. See, also, Edward Carpenter, 'The smoke plague and its remedy', *Macmillan's Magazine*, lxii, 206.

66. On this issue see the comments of Lords Stratheden and Campbell in *Hansard Parliamentary Debates (HL)*, 3rd series, vol. cclxxxviii, 26 May 1884, col. 1, 276–8 and Lord Midleton, ibid., 4th series, i,12 Feb. 1892, col. 301–7. Note also the comments of W. Ewart, 'Medicated air: a suggestion', *Nineteenth Century and After*, lvi (1904), 99. For the context of 'escape' on the part of the social elite see John Premble, *The Mediterranean Passion: Victorians and Edwardians in the South* (Oxford: Oxford University Press, 1988).

67. Douglas Galton, 'On some preventible causes of impurity in London air'. Anniversary Address to the Sanitary Institute, 8 July 1880. See the same author's 'Inaugural address', *Transactions of the Sanitary Institute of Great Britain*, iv (1882–3), 35.

68. Russell, *London Fogs*, 30–1.

69. Stedman Jones, *Outcast London*.

70. *SC Smoke Nuisance*, q. 427, evidence of Ernest Hart.

71. W.D. Hay, *The Doom of the Great City: Being the Narrative of a Survivor Written A. D. 1942* (London: Newman, 1882), 10. Biographical information on Hay is scarce but see the comments by Rosalind Williams in *Notes on the Underground: An Essay on Technology, Society and the Imagination* (Cambridge, Mass.: MIT Press, 1990), 198 and I.F. Clarke, *The Pattern of Expectation 1644–2001* (London: Cape, 1979), 158.

72. Hay, *Doom*, 23.

73. Ibid., 46.

74. Ibid., 49–50.

75. Ibid., 43. The theme of the 'doomed child' loomed large in late nineteenth century degenerationist discourse. See, in this respect, R.C. Ellison, 'On the influence of the purity and impurity of the external air on the health and moral tendencies of a dense population', *Journal of State Medicine*, viii (Feb. 1900), 11.

76. See Raymond Williams, *The Country and the City* (London: Hogarth Press, 1973), ch. 19 and Krishan Kumar, 'Versions of the pastoral: poverty and the poor in English fiction from the 1840s to the 1950s', *Journal of Historical Sociology*, 8 (1995), 1–35.
77. On Gissing see Williams, *Country and City*, 222–5. On Conrad's *Heart of Darkness* (London: Penguin, 1995) see B.Parry, *Conrad and Imperialism: Boundaries and Visionary Fantasies* (London: Macmillan, 1983) and Edward Said, *Culture and Imperialism* (London: Routledge and Kegan Paul, 1978). The latter comments on an 'all-pervading darkness, which by the end of the tale is shown to be the same in London and Africa', 33.
78. Richard Jefferies, *After London or Wild England* (London: Cassell, 1885) and particularly part 1, 'The relapse into barbarism'. The seminal poems by James Thomson are to be found in *City of Dreadful Night* (London: Reeves, 1873): but see also the same author's *Doom of a City* in *The City of Dreadful Night and Other Poems* (London: Reeves, 1880). (Was William Delisle Hay's title borrowed from this source?) In *City of Dreadful Delight: Narratives of Sexual Danger in Late Victorian Britain* (Chicago: University of Chicago Press, 1992), Judith Walkowitz reconstructs the ambience surrounding Conan Doyle's gloomy metropolitan scenarios, and also the visual milieu of two generations of British films set in an ominously fog-ridden East End.
79. F.A.R. (Rollo) Russell, 'The reduction of towns', *Nineteenth Century and After*, li (1902), 131–42.
80. F.A.R. (Rollo) Russell, *Fog and Smoke* (London: P.S. King, 1905), 29.
81. G.B. Longstaff, 'Phthisis, bronchitis and pneumonia: are they epidemic diseases?', *Transactions of the Epidemiological Society of London*, ii (1882–3), 119–28. See also Hardy, *Epidemic Streets*, chs 1 and 8.
82. *Medical Times and Gazette*, ii (1873), 696: *The Lancet*, i (1874), 27–8: *British Medical Journal*, i (1880), 254: and A. Parker, 'Air pollution research and control in Britain', *American Journal of Public Health*, xlvii (1957), 563.
83. Russell, *London Fogs*, 22.
84. See in this respect W.T. Russell, 'The influence of fog on mortality from respiratory diseases', *The Lancet*, ii (1924), 335–9 and the same author's 'The relative influence of fog and low temperature in the mortality from respiratory disease', *The Lancet*, ii (1926), 1128–30.
85. F.J. Brodie, 'Decrease of fog in London during recent years', *Symons Monthly Meteorological Magazine*, xxxix (1904), 213.
86. 'An encouraging feature of the recent fog', *The Lancet*, ii (1899), 183
87. Sir C.A. Cookson, 'A smokeless London', *Journal of State Medicine*, ix (1901), 692. See, also, Brodie, 'Decrease of fog' and Louis C. Parkes, 'The smoke problem in large towns', *Transactions of the Royal Sanitary Institute*, xxviii (1907), 489 and H.T. Bernstein, 'The mysterious disappearance of the Edwardian fog', *The London Journal*, 1 (1978), 189–206.
88. *Sixty Ninth Report of the Registrar-General* (London, HMSO, 1906), cxxxviii.
89. *Seventy First Annual Report of the Registrar-General* (London, HMSO, 1910), cv.

90. *British Medical Journal*, i (1914), 500.

91. H. Heimann, 'Effects of air pollution on human health' in *Air Pollution* (Geneva: World Health Organization, Monograph Series, xlvi, 1961), 176.

92. Simon Szreter, 'The GRO and the public health movement in Britain, 1837–1914', *Social History of Medicine*, 3 (1991), 457–8.

93. Crichton Browne, 'The dust problem', 217.

Chapter 8   Unending Debate: Town, Country and the Construction of the Rural in England, 1870–2000

1. The major conceptual issues are spelt out in M.J. Elson, *Greenbelts: Conflict and Mediation in the Urban Fringe* (London: Heinemann, 1986).

2. See the seminal interwar preservationist polemic, Clough Williams Ellis, *England and the Octopus* (London: Geoffrey Bles, 1928). A decade later, Ellis edited a companion volume on the same theme and called it *Britain and the Beast* (London: J.M. Dent, 1938).

3. Gerald Dix, 'Patrick Abercrombie 1879–1957' in Gordon E. Cherry (ed.), *Pioneers in British Planning* (London: Architectural Press, 1981), 103–30.

4. Peter Hall *et al.*, *The Containment of Urban England: Volume Two: The Planning System* (London: Allen and Unwin, 1973), 73.

5. Peter Hall, *Cities of Tomorrow, An Intellectual History of Urban Planning and Design in the Twentieth Century* (Oxford: Blackwell, 1996), 185 and 333.

6. M.J. Elson *et al.*, *Green Belts and Affordable Housing. Can We Have Both ?* (Bristol: Policy Press, 1996).

7. The aims of the organization are succinctly described at *http://www.countryside-alliance.org.*

8. See, for example, Lawrence Stone, *The Crisis of the Aristocracy* (Oxford: Oxford University Press, 1965), 386–96: Raymond Williams, *The Country and the City* (London: Hogarth Press, 1973) and P.J. Corfield, *The Impact of English Towns 1700–1800* (Oxford: Oxford University Press, 1982), ch. 8.

9. See, in particular, Frank Kermode, *Shakespeare's Language* (London: Penguin Books, 2000), 78–81: Max Byrd, *London Transform'd: Images of the City in the Eighteenth Century* (New Haven and London: Yale University Press, 1978): Jonathan Bate, *Romantic Ecology: Wordsworth and the Environmental Tradition* (London: Routledge, 1991 and Alan Robinson, *Imagining London, 1770–1900* (London: Palgrave, 2005).

10. See, for example, D.H. Lawrence, 'Nottingham and the mining countryside' in E.D. McDonald (ed.), *Phoenix, The Posthumous Papers of D.H. Lawrence* (London: Heinemann, 1961), 133–40 and E.M. Forster, 'The machine stops' in E.M. Forster, *The Collected Short Stories* (London: Sidgwick and Jackson, 1947), 115–50. The same author's *Howard's End* (London: Edward Arnold, 1947), is overwhelmingly preoccupied with the social and relational implications of urban-technological change.

11. Robert Crawford, *The Savage and the City in the Work of T.S. Eliot* (Oxford: Clarendon Press, 1987).

12. See in particular Wilfrid Mellers, *Vaughan Williams and the Vision of Albion* (London: Pimlico, 1989).

13. Michael Rosenthal, *British Landscape Painting* (Oxford: Phaidon, 1982), 124–78.

14. On the long-term demographic development of London see E.A. Wrigley, 'A simple model of London's importance in changing English society and economy 1650–1750', *Past and Present*, 37 (1967), 44–70: P.J. Waller, *Town, City and Country: England 1850–1914* (Oxford: Oxford University Press, 1983), 24–9 and Patricia Garside, 'London and the home counties' in F.M.L. Thompson (ed.), *The Cambridge Social History of Britain 1750–1950: Volume 1: Regions and Communities* (Cambridge: Cambridge University Press, 1990), 498–501.

15. The pre-eminent example is Adna Ferrin Weber, *The Growth of Cities in the Nineteenth Century: A Study in Statistics* (Ithaca: Cornell University Press, 1963), reprint edition.

16. David J. Owen, *The Government of Victorian London 1855–1889: The Metropolitan Board of Works, the Vestries and the City Corporation* (Cambridge MA: Harvard University Press, 1982), edited by Roy MacLeod; John Davis, *Reforming London: The London Government Problem* (Oxford: Clarendon Press, 1988).

17. Here environmental history interacts with larger historiographical debates about shifting conceptions of England and Britain. See Catherine Hills, *The Origins of the English* (London: Duckworth, 2003); Norman Davies, *The Isles: A History* (London: Macmillan, 2000); Krishan Kumar, *A History of English National Identity* (Cambridge: Cambridge University Press, 2003); and Julia Stapleton, *Sir Arthur Bryant and National History in Twentieth Century Britain* (Lanham MD: Lexington, 2005).

18. See, in particular, Jan Marsh, *Back to the Land: The Pastoral Impulse in England 1880–1914* (London: Quartet Books, 1982); P.C. Gould, *Early Green Politics: Back to Nature, Back to the Land and Socialism in Britain, 1880–1900* (Brighton: Harvester Press, 1988); and Dennis Hardy, *Alternative Communities in Nineteenth Century England* (London: Longmans,1979).

19. For comprehensive bibliographical guidance on these much debated issues see Dan Stone, *Breeding Supermen: Nietzsche, Race and Eugenics in Interwar Britain* (Liverpool: Liverpool University Press, 2002); and Mike Hawkins, *Social Darwinism in Europe and America 1860–1945: Nature as Model and Nature as Threat* (Cambridge: Cambridge University Press, 1997).

20. For a penetrating overview see E.J.T. Collins, 'Rural and agricultural change' in Joan Thirsk (ed.), *The Agrarian History of England and Wales. Volume 7, Part 1 1850–1914* (Cambridge: Cambridge University Press, 2000), 138–207.

21. Dudley Baines, *Migration and the Mature Economy: Emigration and Internal Migration in England and Wales 1861–1900* (Cambridge: Cambridge University Press, 1985) and Charlotte Erickson, *Invisible Immigrants: The Adaptation of*

English and Scottish Immigrants in Nineteenth Century America (London: Weidenfeld and Nicolson, 1972).

22. Ideological and party political structures during this period are expertly summarized by K. Theodore Hoppen, *The Mid-Victorian Generation 1846–1886* (Oxford: Oxford University Press, 1998), 131–40 and 638–54 and G.R. Searle, *A New England: Peace and War 1886–1914* (Oxford: Oxford University Press, 2004), ch. 4.

23. Andrew Lees, *Cities Perceived: Urban Society in European and American Thought 1820–1940* (Manchester: Manchester University Press, 1985), part 1.

24. N.G. Harte, (ed.), *The Study of Economic History: Collected Inaugural Lectures, 1893–1970* (London: Cass, 1971), xx. See, also, David Cannadine, 'The present and the past in the English industrial revolution', *Past and Present* 103 (1984), 131–72 and Pat Hudson, *The Industrial Revolution* (London: Edward Arnold, 1992).

25. The key works are J.L. and B.Hammond, *The Town Labourer 1760–1832: The New Civilization* (London: Longmans, Green, 1917); *The Rise of Modern Industry* (London: Methuen, 1925); and *The Village Labourer: A Study in the Government of England before the Reform Bill* (London: Longmans, 1928). For incisive historiographical analysis see R.M. Hartwell, 'The rise of modern industry' in his *The Industrial Revolution and Economic Growth* (London: Methuen, 1971), 81–108.

26. G.M. Trevelyan, *English Social History: A Survey of Six Centuries: Chaucer to Queen Victoria* (London: Longman, 1942).

27. E.P. Thompson, *The Making of the English Working Class* (London: Gollancz, 1963).

28. Each of these writers contributed to Williams Ellis, *Britain and the Beast.*

29. There were similarities between Lawrence's position and the even more extreme stance adopted by Oswald Spengler in his astonishingly vitriolic denunciation of the city, *The Decline of the West* (London: Allen and Unwin, 1932). On the larger issue of elite attitudes towards the proper ends of leisure during this period see D.L. LeMahieu, *A Culture for Democracy: Mass Mind in Britain between the Wars* (Oxford: Oxford University Press, 1988), 103–120 and John Carey, *The Intellectuals and the Masses: Pride and Prejudice among the Literary Intelligentsia 1880–1939* (London: Faber, 1992). See, also, H. Caygill, *Walter Benjamin: The Colour of Experience* (London: Routledge, 1998), ch.3.

30. G.M. Trevelyan, *Must England's Beauty Perish ? A Plea on Behalf of the National Trust for Places of Historic Interest and Natural Beauty* (London: Faber and Dwyer, 1929) and 'Amenities and the state', in Williams Ellis, *Beauty and the Beast*, 183–6. For a scintillating account of the great historian-preservationist's intellectual development see David Cannadine, *G.M. Trevelyan: A Life in History* (London: HarperCollins, 1997).

31. Patrick Abercrombie, *Town and Country Planning* (London: Thornton Butterworth, 1933) and Abercrombie, *Planning in Town and Country: Difficulties and Possibilities* (Liverpool and London: University of Liverpool Press, 1937).

32. See Dennis Hardy, *From Garden Cities to New Towns: Campaigning for Town and Country Planning 1899–1946* (London: Chapman and Hall, 1991).

33. David Matless, *Landscape and Englishness* (London: Reaktion Books, 1998).

34. Valentine Cunningham, *British Writers of the Thirties* (Oxford: Oxford University Press, 1988), 229–38. The case of Baldwin is intriguingly interrogated in Philip Williamson, *Stanley Baldwin: Conservative Leadership and National Values* (Cambridge: Cambridge University Press, 1999). See, also, J. M. Winter, *Sites of Memory, Sites of Mourning: The Great War in English Cultural History* (Cambridge: Cambridge University Press, 1995).

35. R.M. Davis, *Brideshead Revisited: The Past Redeemed* (Boston Mass.: Twayne), 1990.

36. On Hartley there is A.Wright, *Foreign Country: The Life of L.P. Hartley* (London: Andre Deutsch, 1996). See, also, D.P. Vannatta, *H.E. Bates* (Boston Mass.: Twayne, 1983); and Laurie Lee, *Cider with Rosie* (London: Longman, 1967) and *As I Walked Out One Midsummer Morning* (London: Andre Deutsch, 1969).

37. Paul Addison, *The Road to 1945: British Politics in the Second World War* (London: Cape, 1975).

38. Alison Ravetz, *Remaking Cities: Contradictions of the Recent Urban Environment* (London: Croom Helm, 1980), 19–24.

39. P. Richmond, *Marketing Modernisms; The Architecture and Influence of Charles Reilly* (Liverpool: University of Liverpool Press, 2001), 177–98. See, also, Mark Clapson, *Invincible Green Suburbs, Brave New Towns: Social Change and Urban Dispersal in Interwar Britain* (Manchester: Manchester University Press, 1998) and S. Fielding, P. Thompson and N. Tiratsoo, *England Arise! The Labour Party and Popular Politics in 1940s Britain* (Manchester: Manchester University Press, 1985), 102–34.

40. Bill Luckin, 'History, community and utopia: the Manchester reconstruction plan', in Elena Cogato Lanza and Patrizia Bonifazio (eds), *Les Experts de la Reconstruction: Figures et Strategies d'Elite Technique dans L'Europe de L'Apres-Guerre*, (Geneva: MetisPresses, 2009), 37–48.

41. B.W. Clapp, *An Environmental History of the Britain since the Industrial Revolution* (London: Longman,1994), ch. 6.

42. J.B. Thompson, *Ideology and Modern Culture: Critical Social Theory in the Era of Mass Communication* (Cambridge: Cambridge University Press, 1990).

43. Phil Jones, 'The suburban high flat in the post-war reconstruction of Birmingham, 1945–70', *Urban History*, 32 (2005), 308–10.

44. David R. Green, *From Artisans to Paupers: Economic Change and Poverty in London 1780–1870* (Aldershot: Scolar Press, 1995). 'Dishousing' is discussed in J.R. Kellett, *The Impact of the Railways on Victorian Cities* (London: Routledge and Kegan Paul, 1969) and Gareth Stedman Jones, *Outcast London: A Study in the Relationship between Classes in Victorian Society* (Oxford: Oxford University Press, 1971). On the complex balance between low income and rent see E.H. Hunt, *Regional Wage Variations in Britain, 1850–1914* (Oxford: Oxford University Press, 1973).

45. F.M.L. Thompson, 'Introduction' in Thompson (ed.), *The Rise of Suburbia*, (Leicester: Leicester University Press, 1982), 2.

46. F.M.L. Thompson, *Hampstead: Building a Borough, 1650–1954* (London: Routledge Kegan Paul, 1974). See, also, Jane Austen, *Emma* (Harmondsworth: Penguin Books, 1980).

47. This issue has been succinctly summarized by Hoppen, *Mid-Victorian Generation*, 72–90.

48. New perspectives on the issue of health have been opened up by Naomi Williams, 'Death in its season; class, environment and the mortality of infants in nineteenth century Sheffield', *Social History of Medicine*, 5 (1992), 71–94.

49. Thompson, 'Introduction', 6.

50. S.R. Szreter and G.M. Mooney, 'Urbanization, mortality and the standard of living debate: new estimates of expectation of life at birth in nineteenth century British cities', *Economic History Review*, lx (1998), 108–110.

51. See H.J. Dyos and D.A. Reeder, 'Slums and suburbs' in H.J. Dyos and Michael Wolff (eds), *The Victorian City: Images and Realities: Volume 1*, 359–88 and Richard Dennis, 'Modern London' in Martin Daunton (ed.), *Cambridge Urban History of Britain: Volume 3: 1840–1950* (Cambridge: Cambridge University Press, 2000), 117–21.

52. The narrative of Mancunian suburban absorption is related in A. Redford assisted by I.S. Russell, *The History of Local Government in Manchester: Volume 2: Borough and City* (London: Longmans, 1940), 322. For the startling statistics of owner-occupation in England and Wales between the Edwardian period and 1961 see Colin Pooley, 'Patterns on the ground: urban form, residential structure and the social construction of space' in Daunton, *Cambridge Urban History: Vol. 3*, 445.

53. The major contemporary authority on the inter-war slum was the Mancunian and National Liberal politician and businessman, E.D. Simon. See E.D. Simon, *How to Abolish the Slums* (London: Longmans, Green, 1929), *The Anti-Slum Campaign* (London: Longmans, Green, 1933) and *The Rebuilding of Britain: A Twenty Year Plan* (London: Gollancz, 1942). See, in addition, Robert Roberts, *The Classic Slum: Salford Life in the First Quarter of the Century* (Manchester: Manchester University Press, 1971).

54. See the exemplary A. Olechnowicz, *Working-Class Housing in England between the Wars: The Becontree Estate* (Oxford: Oxford University Press, 1997).

55. See James Winter, *Secure from Rash Assault: Sustaining the Victorian Environment* (Berkeley: University of California Press, 1999), 152–61 and R.H. Trainor, *Authority and Social Structure in an Industrial Area: A Study of Three Black Country Towns* (Oxford: Oxford University Press, 1981).

56. The seminal study of a specific area remains H.J. Dyos, *Victorian Suburb: A Study of the Growth of Camberwell* (Leicester: Leicester University Press, 1961).

57. Asa Briggs, *Victorian Cities* (London: Odham's Press, 1963).

58. Carey, *Intellectuals and Masses*, ch. 3.

59. James Winter, *London's Teeming Streets 1830–1914* (London: Routledge, 1993), provides a compelling overview of the hustle and bustle of the nineteenth century capital. However, a group of privileged upper middle-class inhabitants of the metropolis actively campaigned against the hubbub of the street. See John M. Picker, 'The sound-proof study: urban professionals, work space and urban noise', *Victorian Studies*, 42 (1999–2000), 427–53.

60. From the early years of the nineteenth century onwards well-to-do suburbanites were well provided with advice literature on how to import elements of nature into the city. The pioneer was John Claudius Loudon, editor of the *Gardener's Magazine*, and author of *The Suburban Gardener and Villa Companion* (London, 1838) and *The Suburban Horticulturalist* (London, 1842). Both these books were privately published. See Melanie Louise Simo, *Loudon and Landscape: From Country Seat to Metropolis 1783–1943* (New Haven: Yale University Press, 1988).

61. Comparisons between major English and Scottish urban centres will be central to this task. For Scotland see Richard Rodger, *Edinburgh and the Transformation of the Nineteenth Century City: Land, Property and Trust* (New York and Oxford: Oxford University Press, 2000).

Chapter 9   Environmental Justice, History and the City: The United States and Britain, 1970–2000

1. The European dimension should not, of course, be excluded from a survey of this kind. In this respect, a credible case can be made for arguing that, in terms of distinctive national style, the sub-discipline is making more rapid progress in Germany, Scandinavia and France than in Britain. For the evolution of the European discipline as a whole see, successively, Peter L. Brimblecombe and Christian Pfister (eds), *Silent Countdown: Essays in European Environmental History* (London and Berlin: Springer-Verlag, 1990): Dieter Schott (ed.), *Energy and the City in Europe; From the Preindustrial Wood Shortage to the Oil Crisis of the 1970s* (Stuttgart: F. Steiner, 1997); Christian Bernhardt (ed.), *Environmental Problems in European Cities in the Nineteenth and Twentieth Centuries* (Munster and New York: Waxmann, 2001); G. Massard-Guilbaud, H.L. Platt and D. Schott (eds), *Cities and Catastrophes: Coping with Emergency in European History* (Frankfurt am Main, Berlin and New York: Peter Lang, 2002) and C. Bernhardt and G. Massard-Guilbaud (eds), *The Modern Demon: Pollution in Urban and Industrial Societies* (Clermont-Ferrand: Presses Universitaires Blaise-Pascal, 2002).

2. R.J. Evans, *In Defence of History* (London: Granta Books, 1997), provides a succinct overview, albeit from a predominantly 'conservative' perspective, of the great debates within the historical mainstream between the 1970s and the near-present.

3. See here Donald Worster, 'Transformations of the earth: towards an agroecological perspective in history', *Journal of American History*, 76 (1989),

1087–1100; Martin V. Melosi, 'The place of the city in environmental history', *Environmental History Review,* 17 (1993), 1–23: C.M. Rosen and J.A. Tarr, 'The importance of an urban perspective in environmental history', *Journal of Urban History,* 20 (1994), 299–310: W. Cronon, 'A place for stories: nature, history and narrative', *Journal of American History,* 78 (1991–92), 1347–76. These debates have been critically evaluated in Bill Luckin, 'Varieties of the environmental', *Journal of Urban History,* 24 (1997–98), 510–23.

4. There is now a massive literature on the definition, strengths and weaknesses of the concept of environmental justice, but see within the present context Martin V. Melosi, 'Equity, eco-racism and environmental history', *Environmental History Review,* 19 (1995), 1–16 and the same author's 'Environmental justice, political agenda setting, and the myths of history', in Melosi, *Effluent America: Cities, Industry, Energy and the Environment* (Pittsburgh: University of Pittsburgh Press, 2001), 238–62. A creatively sceptical account is provided by C.H. Foreman Jr., *The Promise and Peril of Environmental Justice* (Washington, DC: Brookings Institute, 1998). Comprehensive theoretical overviews include David Harvey, *Justice, Nature and the Geography of Difference* (Oxford: Blackwell, 1996), Part 4 and R. Brulle (ed.), *Agency, Democracy and Nature: The U.S Environmental Movement from a Critical Theory Perspective* (Cambridge, MA. and London: MIT Press, 2000).

5. Dolores Greenberg, 'Reconstructing race and protest: environmental justice in New York City', *Environmental History,* 5 (2000), 223–5. On eco-racism, see R. D. Bullard, *Dumping in Dixie: Race, Class and Environmental Quality* (Boulder, Colorado: Westview Press, 1990): R.D. Bullard (ed.), *Unequal Protection: Environmental Justice and Communities of Colour* (San Francisco: Sierra Club Books, 1994); and A. Szasz, *Ecopopulism: Toxic Waste and the Movement for Environmental Justice* (Minneapolis: University of Minneapolis Press, 1994).

6. Harold L. Platt, 'Jane Addams and the ward boss revisited: class, politics and public health in Chicago, 1890–1930', *Environmental History,* 5 (2000), 194–222. See also the same author's *Shock Cities: The Environmental Transformation and Reform of Manchester and Chicago* (Chicago: University of Chicago Press, 2005).

7. See in particular B.W. Clapp, *An Environmental History of Britain since the Industrial Revolution* (London: Longman, 1994); T.C. Smout, *Nature Contested: Environmental History in Scotland and North England since 1600* (Edinburgh: University of Edinburgh Press, 2000); and John Sheail, *An Environmental History of Twentieth Century Britain* (Basingstoke: Palgrave, 2002). It should, however, be noted that urban-industrialism necessarily constitutes a relatively minor theme in Smout's account. Sheail's study comprises a series of linked case-studies heavily influenced by administrative concerns. In many respects Stephen Mosley, *The Chimney of the World: A History of Smoke Pollution in Victorian and Edwardian Manchester* (Cambridge: White Horse Press, 2001) is the most convincing monograph yet published on the urban-environmental fortunes of a single British city during the modern period.

8. See Melosi, 'Equity and eco-racism' and 'Environmental history and political agenda setting'.

9. R.D. Bullard and B. Wright, 'The politics of pollution: implications for the black community', *Phylon* 47 (1986), 71–8.
10. J. Agyeman, 'Constructing environmental (in)justice: transatlantic tales', *Environmental Politics*, 11 (2002), 36.
11. Andrew Dobson, *Justice and the Environment: Concepts of Environmental Sustainability and Dimensions of Social Justice* (Oxford: Oxford University Press, 1998), 23–6. The key contrast is between individual local and potentially politically explosive conflicts associated with immediate urban problems and those centred on global well-being – the supposedly conventional preoccupation of the non-materialist new social movement approach.
12. See Joel A. Tarr, *The Search for the Ultimate Sink: Urban Pollution in Historical Perspective* (Akron, Ohio: University of Akron Press, 1996); Martin V. Melosi, *Garbage in the City: Refuse, Reform and the Environment 1880–1920* (College Station, Texas: Texas A and M University Press, 1981) and the same author's *The Sanitary City: Urban Infrastructure in America from Colonial Times to the Present* (Baltimore: Johns Hopkins University Press, 2000). William Cronon, *Nature's Metropolis: Chicago and the Great West* (New York: Norton, 1991) has already attained classic status both within the environmental historical community and the disciplinary mainstream.
13. The starting-point for this historiographical tendency was Carolyn Merchant, *The Death of Nature: Women, Ecology and the Scientific Revolution* (London: Wildwood House, 1981). See also Susan M. Hoy 'Municipal housekeeping: the role of women in improving urban sanitation practices', in Martin V. Melosi (ed.), *Pollution and Reform in American Cities* (Austin, Texas: University of Texas Press, 1980), 173–98: Maureen Flanagan, '"The city profitable, the city liveable": environmental policy, gender and power in Chicago in the 1910s', *Journal of Urban History*, 22 (1991), 163–90: Angela Gugliotta, 'Class, gender, and coal smoke: gender, ideology and environmental justice', *Environmental History*, 5 (2000), 165–93; and H.L. Platt, 'Invisible gases: smoke, gender and the redefinition of environmental policy in Chicago 1900–1920', *Planning Perspectives*, 10 (1995), 67–97.
14. See, in particular, the works cited in Cronon, 'A place for stories'.
15. However, this should not be interpreted as implying that the major American urban-environmental pioneers in the United States, and particularly Tarr, Cronon and Melosi, turned a blind eye to the issue of the distribution of power in the city.
16. Platt, 'Jane Addams and the ward boss', 195.
17. Ibid.
18. Ibid., 208.
19. Ibid., 213.
20. Greenberg, 'Reconstructing race and protest', 223.
21. Ibid., 224.
22. Ibid., 225.
23. Ibid.
24. Ibid., 235.

25. Ibid., 239.

26. Ibid., 224.

27. Andrew W. Hurley, *Environmental Inequalities Class, Race and Industrial Pollution in Gary, Indiana 1945–1980* (Chapel Hill and London: University of North Carolina Press, 1995). See the same author's 'Fiasco at Wagner Electric: environmental justice and urban geography in St Louis', *Environmental History*, 4 (1997), 462–3. Greenberg criticizes Hurley for adopting a model which 'rejects the centrality of race' in favour of an interpretation focusing intensively on 'housing opportunities and political disempowerment'. See Greenberg, 'Reconstructing race and protest', 224.

28. Hurley, *Class, Race, and Industrial Pollution*.

29. For an important study of the interwar origins of this idiosyncratic collective *mentalite* see David Matless, *Landscape and Englishness* (London: Reaktion Books, 1998).

30. Frank Perkin, *Middle-Class Radicalism: The Social Bases of the British Campaign for Nuclear Disarmament* (Manchester: Manchester University Press, 1968); Paul Byrne, *The Campaign for Nuclear Disarmament* (London: Croom Helm, 1988) and Ian Welsh, *Mobilising Modernity: The Nuclear Movement* (London: Routledge, 2000).

31. See Michael Brown *et al.*, *The Greenpeace Story* (London: Dorling Kindersley, 1991) and Paul Byrne, *Social Movements in Britain* (London: Routledge, 1997).

32. C. Church, 'The quiet revolution: 10 years since Agenda 21. Measuring the impact of community-based sustained development in the UK. Shell Better Britain Campaign', http:// *www.sbbco.co.uk/reports*. It should be noted that the exceptionally low incomes cited for the poorest sectors of the urban communities cited in this paragraph clearly exclude individual and family state benefits.

33. Ibid.

34. Ibid.

35. Christopher Rootes, 'Environmental protest in Britain, 1988–1997', in B. Seel, M. Paterson and B. Doherty (eds), *Direct Action in British Environmental Protest* (London: Routledge, 2000), 34.

36. However within the social scientific community precisely the converse appears to have been the case, See, for example, Christopher Freeman and Marie Jahoda, (eds), *World Futures: The Great Debate* (London: Martin Robinson, 1978).

37. Many of these texts have adopted a wide-lens *longue duree* approach. See, for example, I.G. Simmons, *An Environmental History of Britain: From 10,000 Years Ago to the Present* (Edinburgh: Edinburgh University Press, 2001). For a representative example of activist-ecological history, see Clive Ponting, *Green History of the World* (London: Sinclair-Stevenson, 1992).

38. Keith Thomas, *Religion and the Decline of Magic: Studies in Popular Beliefs in Sixteenth and Seventeenth Century England* (London: Weidenfeld and Nicolson, 1971) and the same author's *Man and the Natural World: Changing Attitudes in England 1500–1800* (London: Allen Lane Press, 1984). See, also, among a cluster of books concerned with the 'nature of nature', Peter Coates, *Nature:*

238   NOTES TO PAGES 167–168

Western Attitudes since Ancient Times (London: Polity Press, 1998). Keith
Thomas's general approach was brilliantly extended into the nineteenth century
by James Obelkevich, *Religion and Rural Society: South Lindsey, 1825–1875*
(Oxford: Oxford University Press, 1976).

39. The seminal texts underlying the 'two cultures' debate were C.P. Snow, *The Two
    Cultures and the Scientific Revolution* (Cambridge: Cambridge University Press,
    1959) and F.R. Leavis, *Two Cultures: The Significance of C.P. Snow* (London:
    Chatto and Windus, 1962).

40. G.N. von Tunzelmann, 'Trends in real wages 1700–1850, revisited', *Economic
    History Review*, 32 (1979), 49.

41. Key aspects of the urban sector would in due course be investigated by A.S.
    Wohl, *Endangered Lives: Public Health in Victorian Britain* (London: Dent, 1983)
    and John Hassan, *A History of Water in Modern England and Wales* (Manchester:
    Manchester University Press, 1998). See also for studies of individual cities,
    Mosley, *Chimney of the World* and Bill Luckin, *Pollution and Control: A Social
    History of the Thames in the Nineteenth Century* (Bristol and Boston: Adam Hilger,
    1986). Revealingly, and very much in line with the thrust of the general
    argument presented in this chapter, important British urban environmental
    studies have also been published by American historians. Pre-eminent among
    these is Christopher Hamlin, *Public Health and Social Justice in the Age of
    Chadwick: Britain, 1800–54* (Cambridge: Cambridge University Press, 1998).
    But see also D.H. Porter, *The Thames Embankment: Environment, Technology and
    Society in Victorian London* (Akron, Ohio: University of Akron Press, 1998). The
    extent to which Hamlin's conception of 'justice' within a nineteenth century
    urban context coincides with or diverges from contemporary American activist
    definitions is an intriguing issue.

42. See Robert Woods and John Woodward (eds), *Urban Disease and Mortality in
    Nineteenth Century England* (London: Batsford, 1984); Robert Woods and,
    Nicola Shelton, *An Atlas of Victorian Mortality* (Liverpool: University of
    Liverpool Press, 1997); and Robert Woods, *The Demography of Victorian England
    and Wales* (Cambridge: Cambridge University Press, 2000).

43. For incisive bibliographical orientation see Anne Hardy and Simon Szreter,
    'Urban fertility and mortality patterns', in Daunton, *Cambridge Urban History,
    Volume 3*, 637–9. Naomi Williams, 'Death in its season: class, environment and
    the mortality of infant in nineteenth century Sheffield', *Social History of
    Medicine*, 5 (1992), 71–94 proved to be a ground-breaking study.

44. A key institutional factor here has undoubtedly been the very significant
    support given to these sub-disciplines by the highly influential Wellcome
    Trust, which is by far the largest grant-giving body of its kind in Europe.

45. Rootes, 'Environmental protest in Britain'.

46. Agyeman, 'Constructing environmental (in)justice'. However, it cannot be too
    strongly emphasized that sometimes openly, sometimes at a subterranean level,
    racism – and particularly the much discussed phenomenon of 'institutional
    racism' – is alive and kicking in the United Kingdom. Precisely how this

problem should be defined and related to explicitly urban, environmental and historical contexts lies outside the scope of this chapter.

Chapter 10   Place, Disease and Quality of Life in Urban Britain, 1800–1950

1. B.R. Mitchell, *International Historical Statistics: Europe 1750–2000* (Basing-stoke: Palgrave, 2003), Table A4, 74–5 and, throughout this chapter, the classic Adna Ferrin Weber, *The Growth of Cities in the Nineteenth: A Study in Statistics* (London: Macmillan, 1899), 40–56.

2. Geoffrey Best, *Mid-Victorian Britain 1851–75* (London: Weidenfeld and Nicolson, 1971), 11.

3. T. Chandler and G. Fox, *Three Thousand Years of Urban Growth* (New York: Academic Press, 1974), 227.

4. John Langton, 'Urban growth and economic change: from the late seventeenth century to 1841' in Peter Clark (ed.), *Cambridge Urban History of Britain: Volume Two: 1540–1840* (Cambridge: Cambridge University Press, 2000), 453–91.

5. Alan Armstrong, *Stability and Change in an English County Town: A Social Study of York 1801–1851* (Cambridge: Cambridge University Press, 1974), 77.

6. F.M.L. Thompson, 'Town and city' in F.M.L. Thompson (ed.), *The Cambridge Social History of Britain. Volume 1: 1750–1850* (Cambridge: Cambridge University Press, 1990), 8.

7. Simon Szreter and Anne Hardy, 'Urban fertility and mortality patterns' in Martin Daunton (ed.), *The Cambridge Urban History of Britain. Volume 3. 1840–1950* (Cambridge: Cambridge University Press, 2000), 652–5.

8. However, definitions – what constituted a 'town' – complicate the issue. Compare, for example, Jan de Vries, *European Urbanization 1500–1800* (London: Methuen, 1984), 45, Table 3.8 with Paul M. Hohenberg and Lynn Hollen Lees, *The Making of Urban Europe 1000–1950* (Cambridge Mass.: Harvard University Press, 1985), 219, Figure 7.2 and Thompson, 'Town and city', 13, fn. 13. De Vries's '10,000' definition implies a less highly urbanized nation in 1851 than other sources.

9. Andre Armanegaud, 'Population in Europe' in Carlo Cipolla (ed.), *The Fontana Economic History of Europe: The Industrial Revolution* (London: Collins, 1973), 33.

10. E.A. Wrigley, 'A simple model of London's importance in changing English society and economy 1650–1750', *Past and Present*, 37 (1967), 44–70. For a more recent overview see Jeremy Boulton, 'London 1540–1740' in Clark, *The Cambridge Urban History of Britain: Volume Two* (Cambridge, 2000), 315–47.

11. For a perceptive historiographical discussion of Briggs's classic phrase see Harold L. Platt, *Shock Cities: The Environmental Transformation and Reform of Manchester and Chicago* (Chicago: University of Chicago Press, 2005), 15–18.

The theme was originally developed in Asa Briggs, *Victorian Cities* (London: Odham's Press, 1964), ch. 3.

12. Jim Dyos made this point to me in a conversation in the early 1970s.

13. Mitchell, *International Historical Statistics*, Table 4A, 74–5.

14. *Annual* and *Decennial Reports of the Registrar-General*.

15. For the development of Croydon in the nineteenth century see R.C.W. Cox, 'The old centre of Croydon: Victorian decay and development' in A. Everitt (ed.), *Perspectives in Urban History* (London: Macmillan, 1973), 184–212: Nicholas Goddard, '*Sanitate crescamus*: water supply, sewage disposal and environmental values in a Victorian suburb' in Dieter Schott, Bill Luckin and Genevieve Massard-Guilbaud (eds), *Resources of the City: Contributions to an Environmental History of Modern Europe* (Aldershot: Ashgate, 2005), 132–48 and Brian Lancaster, *The 'Croydon Case': Dirty Old Town to Model Town: The Making of the Croydon Board of Health and the Croydon Typhoid Epidemic of 1852–3*, Croydon *Natural History and Scientific Society*, 18 (2001), 145–206.

16. William Cobbett, *Rural Rides; Volume 1*, edited by Asa Briggs (London: Everyman, 1967), 65–6.

17. Andrew Lees, *Cities Perceived; Urban Society in European and American Thought, 1820–1940* (Manchester: Manchester University Press, 1985), part 1 and Richard Dennis, *English Industrial Cities of the Nineteenth Century: A Social Geography* (Cambridge: Cambridge University Press, 1984), 48–109. On changing conceptions of urban catastrophe and collapse in the past see Joe N. Hays, 'Disease as urban disaster: ambiguities and continuities' in Genevieve Massard-Guilbaud, Harold L. Platt and Dieter Schott (eds), *Cities and Catastrophes: Coping with Emergency in European History* (Peter Lang: Oxford, 2002), 63–82. See, also, Simon Szreter, 'Economic growth, disruption, deprivation and death: on the importance of the politics of public health for development' in Szreter, *Health and Wealth: Studies in History and Policy* (Rochester NY: University of Rochester Press, 2005), 203–41 and J.G. Williamson, *Coping with City Growth during the British Industrial Revolution* (Cambridge: Cambridge University Press, 1990).

18. Roderick Floud, Kenneth Wachter and Annabel Gregory, *Height, Health and History: Nutritional Status in the United Kingdom* (Cambridge: Cambridge University Press), 326.

19. Simon Szreter and Graham Mooney, 'Urbanization, mortality and the standard of living debate: new estimates of the expectation of life at birth in nineteenth century British cities', *Economic History Review*, 51 (1998), 94 and 108.

20. See Stewart A. Weaver, *The Hammonds: A Marriage in History* (Stanford: Stanford University Press, 1997), 128–50.

21. The first epidemic has been authoritatively discussed by Michael Durey, *The Return of the Plague: British Society and the Cholera 1831–2* (Dublin: Gill and Macmillan, 1979). See, also, R.J. Morris, *Cholera 1832: The Social Response to an Epidemic* (London: Croom Helm, 1976). On comparative aspects there are Peter Baldwin, *Contagion and the State in Europe 1830–1930* (Cambridge: Cambridge

University Press, 1990) and Christopher Hamlin, *Cholera: The Biography* (Oxford: Oxford University Press, 2009).

22. However, there are two excellent theses – Gerry Kearns, 'Aspects of cholera and society and space in nineteenth century England and Wales', Ph.D. thesis, University of Cambridge, 1985 and Michael Sigsworth, 'Cholera in the large towns of the West and East Ridings, 1843–1983', Ph.D. thesis, Sheffield Polytechnic, 1991. See, also, G. Kearns, 'Cholera, nuisances and environmental management in Islington, 1830–1855' in W. Bynum and R. Porter (eds), *Living and Dying in London: Medical History Supplement 11* (London: Wellcome Institute for the History of Medicine, 1991), 94–125 and Michael Sigsworth and Michael Worboys, 'The public's view of public health in mid-Victorian Britain', *Urban History*, 21 (1994), 237–50.

23. Asa Briggs, 'Cholera and society', *Past and Present*, 119 (1961), 76–96; Richard Evans, 'Epidemics and revolutions: cholera in nineteenth century Europe', *Past and Present*, 120 (1988), 123–46 and Baldwin, *Contagion and the State*. See also Richard Evans, *Death in Hamburg: Society and Politics in the Cholera Years* (Oxford: Clarendon Press, 1987), ch. 4.

24. Margaret Pelling, *Cholera, Fever and English Medicine 1825–1865* (Oxford: Oxford University Press, 1978).

25. Anne Hardy, '"Famine fever or urban crisis?" Typhus in the Victorian city', *Medical History*, 32 (1988), 401–25.

26. F.B. Smith, *The Retreat of Tuberculosis 1850–1950* (London: Croom Helm, 1988), ch. 1. The complexities of defining the national and regional incidence of the disease – and particularly the extent to which it may have included large numbers of victims of 'general respiratory disease' – are discussed in R.I. Woods, *The Demography of Victorian England and Wales* (Cambridge: Cambridge University Press, 2000), 332–40 and 353.

27. Lancaster, '"The Croydon Case"'.

28. Christopher Hamlin, *Public Health and Social Justice in the Age of Chadwick: Britain, 1800–1854* (Cambridge: Cambridge University Press, 1998), 324.

29. Ibid., 324–32.

30. On Carpenter see Nicholas Cambridge, 'The life and times of Dr Alfred Carpenter', University of London. M.D. thesis, 2002. I am grateful to Dr Cambridge for sending me a copy of his dissertation. See, also, Goddard, *Sanitate Crescamus*.

31. Goddard, *Sanitate Crescamus*, 140.

32. Christopher Hamlin, 'Providence and putrefaction: Victorian sanitarians and the natural theology of health and disease', *Victorian Studies*, 28 (1985), 406–9.

33. Alfred Carpenter, *Some Points in the Physiological and Medical Aspect of Sewage Irrigation* (London: Robert Hardwicke, 1870), 43.

34. Alfred Carpenter, *Preventive Medicine in Relation to Public Health* (London: Simpkin, Marshall, 1877), 296.

35. Hamlin, *Public Health and Social Justice*, 332.

36. On John Snow see Peter Vinten-Johansen *et al.*, *Cholera, Chloroform and the Science of Medicine* (Oxford: Oxford University Press, 2003) and George Davey-Smith, 'Behind the Broad Street pump: aetiology, epidemiology, and prevention of cholera in mid-nineteenth century Britain', *International Journal of Epidemiology*, 31 (2002), 920–32. On William Budd see Pelling, *Cholera, Fever and English Medicine*, ch. 7.

37. Christopher Hamlin, 'Edward Frankland's early career as London's official water analyst 1865–1876: the context of "previous sewage contamination"', *Bulletin of the History of Medicine*, 56 (1982), 56–76 and Colin A. Russell, *Edward Frankland: Chemistry, Controversy and Conspiracy in Victorian England* (Cambridge: Cambridge University Press, 1996), 362–97.

38. 'Health of London in 1859' in *Annual Report of the Registrar-General 1859* (London: HMSO, 1860), xxxvii.

39. *Registrar-General's Weekly Returns of Births and Deaths in London*, vol. xxvi, no. 30 cited in *Medical Press and Chronicle*, ii, 1866, 159–60.

40. 'Health of London in 1865' in *Annual Report of the Registrar General 1867* (London: HMSO, 1866), lvii–lviii.

41. Ibid., lvii.

42. See *Sanitary Statistics and Proceedings: Bethnal Green: 1867*, 5–8.

43. 'Scarlet fever', *The Builder*, Oct. 2 1869, 791.

44. *Annual Report of the Medical Officer of Health: Poplar 1869*, 24. See, also, ibid., *Report 1870*, 47.

45. 'The week', *Medical Times and Gazette*, ii, 1869, 464–5.

46. *Annual Report of the Medical Officer of Health 1870: Mile End Old Town*, 23.

47. *Twelfth Annual Report of the Medical Officer to the Privy Council 1870*, British Parliamentary Papers (BPP), 1870, vol. xxxviii, 650.

48. For the origins of the transition see Anne Hardy, 'On the Cusp: Epidemiology and Bacteriology at the Local Government Board, 1890–1905', *Medical History*, 42 (1998), 328–46 and Hardy, '"Exorcizing Molly Malone": typhoid and shellfish consumption in Britain 1860–1960', *History Workshop Journal*, 55 (2003), 73–90. See, also, Jacob Steere-Williams, 'The perfect food and the filth disease: milk-borne typhoid and epidemiological practice in late Victorian Britain', *Journal of the History of Medicine and Allied Sciences*, 65 (2010), 514–45.

49. On the decline of dysentery during the nineteenth century city see Luckin, *Pollution and Control: A Social History of the Thames in the Nineteenth Century* (Bristol and Boston: Adam Hilger, 1986), 101–117.

50. Michael Worboys, *Spreading Germs: Disease Theories and Medical Practice in Britain, 1865–1900* (Cambridge: Cambridge University Press, 2000), 275 and 278.

51. Ibid., 275.

52. See Naomi Williams and Graham Mooney, 'Infant mortality in an "age of great cities": London and the English provincial cities compared', *Continuity and Change*, 9 (1994), 185–212 and Naomi Williams and Chris Galley, 'Urban-rural differentials in infant mortality in Victorian England', *Population Studies*, 49 (1995), 401–20.

53. Hardy, 'On the cusp'.
54. Michael Worboys, *Spreading Germs, passim*. See, also, Michael Worboys, 'Was there a bacteriological revolution in late nineteenth century medicine?, *Studies in the History and Philosophy of Biology and the Biomedical Sciences*, 38 (2007), 20–42.
55. Szreter and Mooney, 'Urbanization, mortality and standard of living', Table 1, 88.
56. See I.S.L. Loudon, 'On maternal mortality, 1900–1960', *Social History of Medicine*, 4 (1991), 29–74 and Loudon, *Death in Childbirth: An International Study of Maternal Care and Maternal Mortality 1800–1950* (Oxford: Oxford University Press, 1992).
57. P. Townsend, N. Davidson and M. Whitehead, *Inequalities in Health: The Black Report* (Harmondsworth: Penguin Books, 1988). See, also, in this context Richard Wilkinson, *Unhealthy Societies: The Afflictions of Inequality* (London: Routledge, 1996), an exceptionally important study for sociologists, historians and policy-makers.
58. *Royal Commission on the Distribution of the Industrial Population: Report* (London: HMSO, 1940), 51–86. See, also, C.H. Lee, 'Regional disparities in infant mortality in Britain, 1871–1971: patterns and hypotheses', *Population Studies*, 45 (1991), 55–65.
59. J.B. Priestley, *English Journey* (London: Heinemann, 1934).
60. E.D. Simon, 'Overcrowding in Didsbury and Ancoats compared', Manchester Central Reference Library, E.D. Simon Papers, M11/16/15, Nov. 21 1919.
61. 'Survey of 1,076 homes in Hulme' in *How Manchester is Managed* (Manchester, 1939), 8.
62. John Stevenson and Chris Cook, *The Slump: Society and Politics during the Depression* (London: Cape, 1977), 285.
63. Lara Marks, *Metropolitan Maternity: Maternal and Infant Welfare Services in Early Twentieth Century London* (Amsterdam and Atlanta: Rodopi, 1996), 98.
64. R.S. Lambert, *Sir John Simon 1816–1904 and English Social Administration* (London: MacGibbon and Kee, 1963), 199; Goddard, *Sanitate Crescamus*, 140.
65. H.L. Murphy, *Report on a Local Inquiry into an Outbreak of Typhoid Fever at Croydon in October and November 1937* (London: HMSO, 1938). See, also, 'Croydon typhoid inquiry: history of the outbreak', *British Medical Journal*, ii, December 25 1937, 1293–5 and 'Safeguarding water supplies', *Nature*, 144, Aug. 12. 1937, 282.
66. D.F. Smith, H.L. Diack and T.H. Pennington, *Food Poisoning, Policy and Politics: Corned Beef and Typhoid in Britain in the 1960s* (Woodbridge: Boydell and Brewer, 2005), 13–14.
67. 'Croydon typhoid inquiry', 1293–5.
68. *County Borough of Croydon: Annual Report of the Medical Officer of Health and School Medical Service for the Year 1945* (Croydon, 1946), 5.
69. *Annual Report of the MoH*, 1946, 78, 82. See, also, *Annual Report of the Medical Officer of Health and Principal School Medical Officer for the Year 1955* (Croydon, 1956), 11.

70. *Annual Report of the MoH 1946*, 82.
71. Ibid. *1945*, 5.
72. Ibid. *1946*, ix.
73. Ibid. *1950*, 5.
74. Ibid.
75. *Annual Report of the MoH 1954*, 3.
76. Ibid. *1953*, 2.
77. Ibid. *1954*, 96–7.

BIBLIOGRAPHY

Abel-Smith, Brian, *The Hospitals, 1800–1948: A Study in Social Administration in England and Wales* (London, 1964).

Abercrombie, Patrick, *Planning in Town and Country: Difficulties and Possibilities* (Liverpool and London, 1937).

Ackerknecht, Erwin Heinz, 'Anticontagionism between 1821 and 1876', *Bulletin of the History of Medicine*, 22 (1948), 562–93.

———, *History and Geography of the Most Important Diseases* (New York, 1965).

Adams, I.H., *The Making of Urban Scotland* (London, 1978).

Addison, Paul, *The Road to 1945: British Politics in the Second World War* (London, 1975).

Agyeman, J., 'Constructing environmental (in)justice: transatlantic tales', *Environmental Politics*, 11 (2002), 31–53.

Amsterdamska, Olga and Hiddinga, Anja, 'Trading zones or citadels? professionalization and intellectual change in the history of medicine', in Frank Huisman and John Harley Warner (ed.), *Locating Medical History: The Stories and their Meanings*, 11–33.

Appleby, Andrew B., 'Disease or famine? Mortality in Cumberland and Westmorland 1580–1640', *Economic History Review*, 26 (1973), 403–33.

———, 'Nutrition and disease: the case of London, 1550–1750', *Journal of Interdisciplinary History*, 6 (1975), 1–22.

———, 'The disappearance of the plague', *Economic History Review*, 33 (1980), 161–73.

Ariès, Philipe, *Western Attitudes Towards Death: From the Middle Ages to the Present* (Baltimore, 1974).

Armegaud, Andre, 'Population in Europe' in Carlo Cipolla (ed.), *The Fontana Economic History of Europe: The Industrial Revolution* (London, 1973), 25–71.

Armstrong, Alan, *Stability and Change in an English County Town: A Social Study of York 1801–1851* (Cambridge, 1974).

Ashby, E., and Anderson, M., 'Studies in the politics of environmental protection: the historical roots of the British Clean Air Act, 1956. II. The ripening of public opinion, 1898–1952', *Interdisciplinary Science Reviews*, 2 (1977), 190–206.

Ashby, Eric and Anderson, Marion, *The Politics of Clean Air* (Oxford, 1981).
Ayers, G.M., *England's First State Hospitals and the Metropolitan Asylums Board, 1867 – 1930* (London, 1971).
Bailes, K.E., *Environmental History: Critical Issues in Comparative Perspective* (Lanham MD, 1985).
Baines, Dudley, *Migration and the Mature Economy: Emigration and Internal Migration in England and Wales 1861 – 1900* (Cambridge, 1985).
Baldwin, Peter, *Contagion and the State in Europe 1830 – 1930* (Cambridge, 1990).
Barber, B.J., 'Aspects of municipal government, 1835 – 1914' in D. Fraser (ed.), *A History of Modern Leeds* (Manchester, 1980), 301 – 26.
Barker, T.C. and J.R. Harris, *A Merseyside Town in the Industrial Revolution* (Liverpool, 1954).
Barnes, David S., 'Confronting sensory crisis in the Great Stinks of London and Paris' in W.A. Cohen and Ryan Johnson, (eds), *Filth: Dirt, Disgust and Modern Life* (Minneapolis, 2005), 529 – 41.
Bartrip, Peter, 'Food for the body and food for the mind: the regulation of freshwater fisheries in the 1870s', *Victorian Studies*, 28 (1985), 285 – 304.
———, '*The British Medical Journal*: a retrospect' in W.F. Bynum, R.S. Porter and Stephen Lock (eds), *Medical Journals and Medical Knowledge* (London,1992), 126 – 45.
Bate, Jonathan, *Romantic Ecology: Wordsworth and the Environmental Tradition* (London, 1991).
Benidickson, Jamie, *The Culture of Flushing: A Social and Legal History of Sewage* (Vancouver, 2007).
Bernhardt, Christoph (ed.), *Environmental Problems in European Cities in the Nineteenth and Twentieth Centuries* (Munster and New York, 2001).
———, and Genevieve Massard-Guilbaud (eds), *The Modern Demon: Pollution in Urban and Industrial European Societies* (Clermont-Ferrand, 2002).
Bernstein, H.T., 'The mysterious disappearance of the Edwardian London fog', *London Journal*, 2 (1975), 189 – 206.
Best, Geoffrey, *Mid-Victorian Britain 1850 – 75* (London, 1971).
Bijker, W.E., T.P. Hughes and T.J. Pinch (eds), *The Social Construction of Technological Systems: New Directions in the Sociology and History of Technology* (Cambridge, 1992).
———, and John Law (eds), *Shaping Technology/Building Society: Studies in Sociotechnical Change* (Cambridge, 1992).
Blackman, Janet, 'Popular theories of generation: the evolution of *Aristotle's Works*. The study of an anachronism', in John Woodward and David Richards (eds), *Health Care and Popular Medicine in Nineteenth Century England* (London, 1977), 56 – 89.
Blake, E.H. and W.R. Jenkins, *Drainage and Sanitation* (London, 1956).
Blake, N.M., *Water for the Cities: A History of the Urban Water Supply Problem in the United States* (New York, 1956).
Bocking, Stephen, 'Environmentalism' in Peter L. Bowler and John V. Pickstone (eds), *The Cambridge History of Science. Volume Six: The Modern Biological and Earth Sciences* (Cambridge, 2009), 602 – 21.

Boon, Tim, 'The smoke menace: cinema, sponsorship and the social relations of science in 1937' in Michael Shortland (ed.), *Science and Nature: Essays in the History of the Environmental Sciences*, (Stanford-in-the-Vale, 1993), 57–87.

Boulton, Jeremy, 'London 1540–1740' in Peter Clark (ed.), *The Cambridge Urban History of Britain: Volume Two* (Cambridge, 2000), 315–47.

Bowler, Catherine and Peter L. Brimblecombe, 'The difficulties of abating smoke in late Victorian York', *Atmospheric Environment*, 24B (1990), 49–55.

Bowler, Peter, L., *The Fontana History of the Environmental Sciences* (London, 1992).

Brantlinger, Patrick. (ed.), *Energy and Entropy: Science and Culture in Victorian Britain: Selected Essays from Victorian Studies* (Bloomington, 1988).

Braudel, Fernand, *Capitalism and Material Life*, translated by M. Kochan (London, 1974).

Brenner, J.F., 'Nuisance law and the industrial revolution', *Journal of Legal Studies*, 3 (1974), 403–33.

Briggs, Asa, 'Cholera and society in the nineteenth century', *Past and Present*, 19 (1961), 79–96.

———, *Victorian Cities* (London, 1963).

———, *Victorian Things* (Harmondsworth, 1990).

Brimblecombe, Peter L., *The Big Smoke: A History of Air Pollution in London since Medieval Times* (London, 1987).

———. and Christian Pfister (eds), *Silent Countdown: Essays in European Environmental History* (London and Berlin, 1990).

Brown, Michael, *et al.*, *The Greenpeace Story* (London, 1991).

Bruce, F.E., 'Water supply and waste disposal', in T.I. Williams (ed.), *A History of Technology, Volume Seven: The Twentieth Century c. 1990 to c. 1950* (Oxford, 1958), 1382–98.

Brulle, R. (ed.), *Agency, Democracy and Nature: The U.S. Environmental Movement from a Critical Theory Perspective* (Cambridge, 2000).

Budge, Ian and C. O'Leary, *Belfast: Approach to Crisis. A Study of Belfast Politics 1613–1970* (London, 1973).

Bullard, R.D., *Dumping in Dixie: Race, Class and Environmental Quality* (Colorado, 1990).

———, (ed.), *Unequal Protection: Environmental Justice and Communities of Color* (San Francisco, 1994).

———, and B. Wright, 'The politics of pollution: implications for the black community', *Phylon*, 47 (1986), 71–8.

Burnet, MacFarlane and David O. White, *The Natural History of Infectious Disease* (Cambridge, 1972).

Burrow, J.W., *Evolution and Society: A Study in Victorian Social Theory* (Cambridge, 1966).

Byrd, Max, *London Transform'd: Images of the City in the Eighteenth Century* (New Haven and London, 1978).

Byrne, Paul, *The Campaign for Nuclear Disarmament* (London, 1988).

———, *Social Movements in Britain* (London, 1997).

Cage, R.A., 'Health in Glasgow' in R.A. Cage (ed.), *The Working-Class in Glasgow* (London 1987), 56–76.

Cambridge, Nicholas, 'The life and times of Dr Alfred Carpenter', University of London, M.D. thesis, 2002.

Cannadine, David, 'The present and the past in the English industrial revolution', *Past and Present*, 103 (1984), 131–72.

———, G.M. *Trevelyan: A Life in History* (London, 1997).

Carey, John, *The Intellectuals and the Masses: Pride and Prejudice among the Literary Intelligentsia 1880–1939* (London, 1992).

Caygill, H., *Walter Benjamin: The Colour of Experience* (London, 1998).

Chambers, J.D., *Population, Economy and Society in Pre-Industrial England* (Oxford, 1972).

Chandler, T.J., *The Climate of London* (London, 1965).

———, and G. Fox, *Three Thousand Years of Urban Growth* (New York, 1974).

Chapman, S.D. (ed.), *The History of Working Class Housing: A Symposium* (Newton Abbott, 1971).

Checkland, O., and M. Lamb (eds), *Health Care as Social History* (Aberdeen, 1982).

Checkland, S.G., *The Rise of Industrial Society in England 1815–1885* (London, 1971).

Chevalier, Louis (ed.), *Le Choléra: La Première Epidémie du XIXe siècle* (La Roche-sur-Yon, 1958).

Church, Chris, *The Quiet Revolution: 10 Years since Agenda 21; Measuring the Impact of Community-based Sustainable Development in the UK* (Birmingham, 2002).

Cipolla, Carlo M., *Cristofano and the Plague: A Study in the History of Public Health in the Age of Galileo* (London, 1973).

———, *Public Health and the Medical Profession in the Renaissance* (Cambridge, 1976).

Clapp, B.W, *An Environmental History of Britain since the Industrial Revolution*, (London, 1994).

Clapson, Mark, *Invincible Green Suburbs, Brave New Towns: Social Change and Urban Dispersal in Interwar Britain* (Manchester, 1998).

Clarke, I.F., *The Pattern of Expectation 1644–2001* (London, 1979).

Clifton, Gloria, *Professionalism, Patronage and Public Service in Victorian London* (London: UCL Press, 1992).

Clinton, A. and P.Murray, 'Reassessing the vestries: London local government, 1855–1900' in A. O'Day (ed.), *Government and Institutions in the Post-1832 United Kingdom* (Lewiston, 1995), 51–84.

Coates, Peter, *Nature: Western Attitudes since Ancient Times* (London, 1998).

Collins, E.J. T., 'Rural and agricultural change' in Joan Thirsk (ed.), *The Agrarian History of England and Wales. Volume 7, Part 1, 1850–1914* (Cambridge, 2000), 138–207.

Condrau, Flurin, 'The Patient Meets the Clinical Gaze', *Social History of Medicine*, 20 (2007), 525–40.

Cooter, Roger, "Framing" the End of the Social History of Medicine' in Huisman, Frank and John Harley Warner (eds), *Locating Medical History: The Stories and their Meanings* (Baltimore, 2004), 309–37.

———, 'After death/after-"life"': the social history of medicine in post-postmodernity', *Social History of Medicine*, 20 (2007), 441–64.

Corbin, A., *The Foul and the Fragrant: Odor and the French Social Imagination* (Leamington Spa, 1986), translated by M. Kochan.

Corfield, P.J., *The Impact of British Towns 1700–1800* (Oxford, 1982).

Cox, R.C. W., 'The old centre of Croydon: Victorian decay and development' in A. Everitt (ed.), *Perspectives in Urban History* (London, 1973), 184–212.

Crawford, Margaret E., 'Typhus in nineteenth century Ireland' in Greta Jones and
  Elizabeth Malcolm (eds), *Medicine, Disease and the State in Ireland 1650–1940*
  (Cork, 1999), 121–37.
Crawford, Robert, *The Savage and the City in the Work of T.S. Eliot* (Oxford, 1987).
Creighton, Charles, *A History of Epidemics in Britain. Two Volumes*, edited by D.E.C.
  Eversley (London, 1965).
Crellin, J.K., 'The dawn of the germ theory: particles, infection and biology' in F.N.
  L. Poynter (ed.), *Science and Medicine in the 1860s* (London, 1968), 57–76.
Cronon, William., 'A place for stories: nature, history and narrative', *Journal of
  American History*, 78 (1991–92), 1347–76.
———, *Nature's Metropolis: Chicago and the Great West* (New York, 1991).
Crook, Tom, 'Sanitary inspection and the public sphere in late Victorian and
  Edwardian Britain: a case study in liberal governance', *Social History*, 32 (2007),
  369–93.
Crosby, A.W., *Ecological Imperialism: The Biological Expansion of Europe 900–1900*
  (Cambridge, 1986).
Cullen, M.J., *The Statistical Movement in Early Victorian Britain* (Hassocks, 1979).
Cunningham, Valentine, *British Writers of the Thirties* (Oxford, 1988).
Daunton, M.J., *House and Home in the Victorian City: Working Class Housing 1850–
  1914* (London, 1983).
Davey-Smith, George, 'Behind the Broad Street pump: aetiology, epidemiology, and
  prevention of cholera in mid-nineteenth century Britain', *International Journal of
  Epidemiology*, 31 (2002), 920–32.
Davies, Norman, *The Isles: A History* (London, 2000).
Davis, John. *Reforming London: The London Government Problem, 1855–1900* (Oxford,
  1988).
Davis, R.M., *Brideshead Revisited: The Past Redeemed* (Boston, 1990).
Davison, Graeme, 'The city as a natural system: theories of urban society in early
  nineteenth-century Britain', in Derek Fraser and Anthony Sutcliffe (eds),
  The Pursuit of Urban History (London, 1983), 349–70.
De Vries, Jan, *European Urbanization 1500–1800* (London, 1984).
Dennis, Richard, *English Industrial Cities of the Nineteenth Century: A Social Geography*
  (Cambridge, 1984), 48–109.
———, 'Modern London' in M. Daunton (ed.), *Cambridge Urban History of Britain
  Volume Three: 1840–1950* (Cambridge, 2000).
Desmond, Adrian, *Huxley: Devil's Disciple to Evolution's High Priest* (London, 1997).
Dingle, A.E. '"The monster nuisance of all": landowners, alkali manufacturers and
  air pollution 1828–1864', *Economic History Review*, 35 (1982), 529–48.
Dix, Gerald, 'Patrick Abercrombie 1879–1957' in Gordon E. Cherry (ed.), *Pioneers
  in British Planning* (London, 1981), 103–30.
Dobson, Andrew, *Justice and the Environment: Concepts of Environmental Sustainability
  and Dimensions of Social Justice* (Oxford, 1998).
Dobson, Mary J., *Contours of Death and Disease in Early Modern England* (Cambridge,
  1997).
Douglas, Mary, *Purity and Danger: An Analysis of Concepts of Pollution and Taboo*
  (London, 1966).
———, 'Environments at risk' in Douglas, *Implicit Meanings: Selected Essays in
  Anthropology* (London, 1975), 230–48.

————, and Aaron Wildavsky, *Risk and Culture: An Essay on the Selection of Technical and Environmental Dangers* (Berkeley and London, 1982).

Durey, Michael, *The First Spasmodic Cholera Epidemic in York, 1832* (York, 1974).

————, *The Return of the Plague: British Society and the Cholera 1831–2* (Dublin, 1979).

Dwork, Deborah, *War is Good for Babies and Other Young Children. A History of the Infant and Child Welfare Movement in England. 1898–1918* (London and New York, 1987).

Dyos, H.J., 'Railways and housing in Victorian London', *Journal of Transport History*, 2 (1955), 11–21.

————, 'Some social costs of railway building in London', *Journal of Transport History*, 3 (1957–8), 23–30.

————, *Victorian Suburb: A Study of the Growth of Camberwell* (Leicester, 1961).

————, and D.A. Reeder, 'Slums and suburbs' in Dyos, H. J. and Michael Wolff (eds), *The Victorian City: Images and Realities.Volume Two* (London, 1978), 359–86.

————, 'Great and Greater London: notes on metropolis and provinces in the nineteenth and twentieth centuries', in David Cannadine and David Reeder (eds), *Exploring the Urban Past: Essays in Urban History by H.J. Dyos* (Cambridge, 1982), 37–55.

Ehrlich, Paul R. and A.H. Ehrlich, *Population, Resources, Environment: Issues in Human Ecology* (San Francisco, 1970).

Elson, Martin J., *Green Belts: Conflict Mediation in the Urban Fringe* (London, 1986).

Elson, M.J. *et al.*, *Green Belts and Affordable Housing. Can We Have Both?* (Bristol, 1996).

Erickson, Charlotte, *Invisible Immigrants: The Adaptation of English and Scottish Immigrants in Nineteenth Century America* (London, 1972).

Evans, Richard J., *Death in Hamburg: Society and Politics in the Cholera Years, 1830–1910* (Oxford, 1987).

————, 'Epidemics and revolutions: cholera in nineteenth century Europe', *Past and Present*, 120 (1988), 123–46.

————, *In Defence of History* (London, 1997).

Eyler, John M., 'William Farr on the cholera: the sanitarian's disease theory and the statistician's method', *Journal of the History of Medicine and Allied Sciences*, 28 (1973), 79–100.

————, *Victorian Social Medicine: The Ideas and Methods of William Farr* (Baltimore, 1979).

————, *Sir Arthur Newsholme and State Medicine 1885–1935* (Cambridge, 1997).

Ferguson, Niall *et al.*, *The Shock of the Global: The 1970s in Perspective* (Cambridge, 2010).

Fielding, Steven, Peter Thompson and Nick Tiratsoo, *England Arise! The Labour Party and Popular Politics in 1940s Britain* (Manchester, 1985).

Finer, S.E., *The Life and Times of Sir Edwin Chadwick* (London, 1952).

Flanagan, Maureen, '"The city profitable, the city liveable": environmental policy, gender and power in Chicago in the 1910s', *Journal of Urban History*, 22 (1991), 163–90.

Flick, Carlos, 'The movement for smoke abatement in nineteenth-century Britain', *Technology and Culture*, 21 (1980), 29–50.

Flinn, M.W. (ed.), *Report on the Sanitary Condition of the Labouring Population of Great Britain by Edwin Chadwick 1842* (Edinburgh, 1965).

————, 'The stabilization of mortality in pre-industrial Europe', *Journal of European Economic History*, 3 (1974), 285–318.

————, 'Plague in Europe and the Mediterranean countries', *Journal of European Economic History*, 8 (1979), 131–48.

————, and T.C. Smout (eds), *Essays in Social History* (Oxford, 1974).

Flintoff, F. and R. Millard, *Public Cleansing* (London, 1969).

Floud, Roderick, Kenneth Wachter and Annabel Gregory, *Height, Health and History: Nutritional Status in the United Kingdom* (Cambridge, 1990).

Foreman, C.H., *The Promise and Peril of Environmental Justice* (Washington, 1998).

Forster, E.M., 'The machine stops' in E.M. Forster, *The Collected Short Stories* (London, 1947), 115–50.

Foucault, Michel, *The Birth of the Clinic: An Archaeology of Medical Perception*. Translated by Alan Sheridan. (London, 1973).

Fraser, Derek, *Urban Politics in Victorian England: The Structure of Politics in Victorian Cities* (Leicester, 1976).

————, *Power and Authority in the Victorian City* (Oxford, 1979).

Freeman, Christopher, and Marie Jahoda (eds), *World Futures: The Great Debate* (London, 1978).

Gandy, Matthew, *Recycling and Waste: An Exploration of Contemporary Environmental Policy* (Aldershot, 1993).

————, *Recycling and the Politics of Urban Waste* (London, 1994).

Garrett, Eilidh *et al.*, *Infant Mortality: A Continuing Social Problem* (Aldershot, 2007).

————, and Alice Reid, '"Satanic mills, pleasant lands": spatial variation in women's work and infant mortality as viewed from the 1911 *Census*', *Historical Research*, 68 (1994), 156–77.

Garside, Patricia, L., 'London and the Home Counties' in F.M.L. Thompson (ed.), *Cambridge Social History of Britain, Volume 1: Regions and Communities* (Cambridge, 1990), 471–539.

Garwood, Christine, 'Green crusaders or captives of industry? The British alkali industry and the ethics of environmental decision-making', *Annals of Science*, 61 (2004), 99–117.

Gibbon, G. and R.W. Bell, *History of the London County Council 1889–1939* (London, 1939).

Gladstone, G.P., 'Pathogenicity and virulence of microorganisms', in Howard Florey (ed.), *General Pathology* (London, 1970).

Glick, T.F., 'Science, technology and the urban environment: the Great Stink of 1858' in L.J. Bilsky (ed.), *Historical Ecology* (Port Washington,1980), 122–39.

Goddard, Nicholas, '"A mine of wealth": the Victorians and the agricultural value of sewage', *Journal of Historical Geography*, 22 (1996), 274–90.

————, '*Sanitate crescamus*: water supply, sewage disposal and environmental values in a Victorian suburb' in Dieter Schott, Bill Luckin and Genevieve Massard-Guilbaud (eds), *Resources of the City: Contributions to an Environmental History of Modern Europe* (Aldershot, 2005), 132–48.

Goodall, E.W., *A Short History of the Infectious Epidemic Diseases* (London, 1934).

Gould, P.C., *Early Green Politics: Back to Nature, Back to the Land and Socialism in Britain, 1880–1900* (Brighton, 1988).

Grant, R.K. J., 'Merthyr Tydfil in the mid-nineteenth century: the struggle for public health', *Welsh History Review*, 14 (1989), 574–94.

Green, David R., *From Artisans to Paupers: Economic Change and Poverty in London 1780–1870* (Aldershot, 1995).

Greenberg, Dolores, 'Reconstructing race and protest: environmental justice in New York City', *Environmental History*, 5 (2000), 223–50.

Greenwood, Major, *Epidemics and Crowd Diseases* (London, 1935).

Gugliotta, Angela, 'Class, gender, and coal smoke: gender, ideology and environmental justice', *Environmental History*, 5 (2000), 165–93.

Hall, Peter *et al.*, *The Containment of Urban England: Volume Two: The Planning System* (London, 1973).

————, *Cities of Tomorrow, An Intellectual History of Urban Planning and Design in the Twentieth Century* (Oxford, 1996).

Halliday, Stephen, *The Great Stink of London: Sir Joseph Bazalgette and the Cleansing of the Victorian Metropolis* (Stroud, 1998).

Hamlin, Christopher, 'Edward Frankland's career as London's official water analyst 1865–1876: the context of "previous sewage contamination"', *Bulletin of the History of Medicine*, 56 (1982), 56–76.

————, 'Providence and putrefaction: Victorian sanitarians and the natural theology of health and disease', *Victorian Studies*, 3 (1985), 381–411.

————, 'William Dibdin and the idea of biological sewage treatment', *Technology and Culture*, 29 (1988), 189–218.

————, 'Muddling in bumbledom: on the enormity of large sanitary improvements in four British towns, 1855–1885', *Victorian Studies*, 33 (1988–9), 55–83.

————, *A Science of Impurity: Water Analysis in Nineteenth Century Britain* (Berkeley, 1990).

————, 'Edwin Chadwick and the engineers, 1842–1854: systems and anti-systems in the pipe-and-brick sewers war', *Technology and Culture*, 33 (1992), 680–709.

————, 'Environmental sensibility in Edinburgh, 1839–40: The "fetid irrigation" controversy', *Journal of Urban History*, 20 (1994), 311–39.

————. *Public Health and Social Justice in the Age of Chadwick: Britain, 1800–1854*, (Cambridge, 1998).

————, 'Public sphere to public health: the transformation of "nuisance"' in Steven Sturdy (ed.), *Medicine, Health and the Public Sphere in Britain, 1600–2000* (London, 2002), 190–204.

————, 'Sanitary policing and the local state, 1873–74: a statistical study of English and Welsh towns', *Social History of Medicine*, 17 (2005), 39–61.

————, 'The city as a chemical system? The chemist as urban environmental professional in France and Britain 1780–1880', *Journal of Urban History*, 33 (2007), 702–28.

————, *Cholera: The Biography* (Oxford, 2009).

Hammond, J.L., 'The industrial revolution and discontent', *Economic History Review*, 1 (1930), 215–28.

Hanley, James G., 'Parliament, physicians and nuisances: the demedicalization of nuisance law, 1831–1855', *Bulletin of the History of Medicine*, 80 (2006), 702–32.

Hardy, Anne, 'Water and the search for public health in London in the eighteenth and nineteenth centuries', *Medical History*, 28 (1984) 250–84.

————, '"Famine fever or urban crisis?" Typhus in the Victorian city', *Medical History*, 32 (1988), 401–25.

————, 'Public health and the expert: the London medical officers of health, 1856–1900' in R.M. MacLeod (ed.), *Government and Expertise: Specialists, Administrators and Professionals, 1860–1919* (Cambridge, 1988), 128–42.

————, 'Parish pump to private pipes: London's water supply in the nineteenth century' in W.F. Bynum and Roy Porter (eds), *Living and Dying in London: Medical History Supplement 11* (London, 1991), 76–93.

————, 'Rickets and the rest: childcare, diet and the infectious children's diseases', *Social History of Medicine*, 5 (1992), 389–412.

————, *The Epidemic Streets: Infectious Disease and the Rise of Preventive Medicine 1856–1900* (Oxford, 1993).

————, 'On the cusp: epidemiology and bacteriology at the Local Government Board, 1890–1905', *Medical History*, 42 (1998), 328–46.

————, '"Exorcizing Molly Malone": typhoid and shellfish consumption in Britain 1860–1960', *History Workshop Journal*, 55 (2003), 73–90.

Hardy, Dennis, *From Garden Cities to New Towns: Campaigning for Town and Country Planning 1899–1946* (London, 1991).

Harris, Bernard, 'Public health, nutrition and the decline of mortality: the McKeown thesis revisited', *Social History of Medicine*, 17 (2004), 379–407.

————, Martin Gorsky, Aravinda Guntupalli and Andrew Hinde, 'Ageing, sickness, and health in England and Wales during the mortality transition', *Social History of Medicine*, 24 (2011), 643–65.

Harris, Jose, *Private Lives, Public Spirit: Britain 1870–1914* (Oxford, 1993).

Harte, N.G. (ed.), *The Study of Economic History: Collected Inaugural Lectures, 1893–1970* (London, 1971).

Hartwell, R.M., *The Industrial Revolution and Economic Growth* (London, 1971).

Harvey, David, *Justice, Nature and the Geography of Difference* (Oxford, 1996).

Hassan, J.A., 'The growth and impact of the British water industry in the nineteenth century', *Economic History Review*, 38 (1985), 531–47.

————, *Prospects for Economic and Environmental History* (Manchester, 1995).

————, 'The water industry, 1900–1951: a failure of public policy?' in Robert Millward and John Singleton (eds), *The Political Economy of Nationalisation in Britain 1920–1950* (Cambridge, 1995).

————, *A History of Water in Modern England and Wales* (Manchester, 1998).

Hawes, Richard, 'The municipal regulation of smoke pollution in Liverpool, 1853–1866', *Environment and History*, 4 (1998), 75–90.

Hawkins, Mike, *Social Darwinism in Europe and America 1860–1945: Nature as Model and Nature as Threat* (Cambridge, 1997).

Hays, Jo N., 'Disease as urban disaster: ambiguities and continuities' in Genevieve Massard-Guilbaud, Harold L. Platt and Dieter Schott (eds), *Cities and Catastrophes: Coping with Emergency in European History* (Oxford, 2002), 63–82.

Helleiner, K.F., 'The population of Europe from the Black Death to the eve of the vital revolution', *Cambridge Economic History of Europe, Volume Four* (Cambridge, 1967), 1–95.

Hennock, E.P., *Fit and Proper Persons: Ideal and Reality in Nineteenth Century Urban Government* (London, 1964).

Henry, Louis, 'The population of France in the eighteenth century' in D.V. Glass and David Eversley (eds), *Population in History* (London, 1965), 449–94.

Higgs, Edward, *Life, Death and Statistics: Civil Registration, Censuses and the Work of the General Register Office* (Hatfield, 2004).

Higgs, R., 'Cycles and trends in mortality in 18 large American cities, 1871–1900', *Explorations in Economic History*, 16 (1979), 381–408.

Hills, Catherine, *The Origins of the English* (London, 2003).

Himmelfarb, Gertrude, *The Idea of Poverty: England in the Early Industrial Age* (New York,1984).

Hobsbawm, E.J., *Labouring Men: Studies in the History of Labour* (London, 1968).

———, 'The British standard of living, 1790–1850' in A.J. Taylor (ed.), *The Standard of Living in Britain in the Industrial Revolution* (London, 1975), 58–92.

Hohenberg, Paul M. and Lynn Hollen Lees, *The Making of Urban Europe 1000–1950* (Cambridge Mass., 1985).

Hoppen, Theodore K., *The Mid-Victorian Generation 1846–1886* (Oxford, 1998).

House, J.W., *North Eastern England: Population Movements and the Landscape since the Early Nineteenth Century* (Durham, 1954).

Hoy, S., '"Municipal housekeeping". The role of women in improving urban sanitation practices, 1880–1917' in Martin Melosi (ed.), *Pollution and Reform in American Cities 1870–1930* (Austin,1980), 173–98.

Hudson, Pat, *The Industrial Revolution* (London, 1992).

Hunt, E.H., *Regional Wage Variations in Britain, 1850–1914* (Oxford, 1973).

Hurley, Andrew W., *Environmental Inequalities: Class, Race and Industrial Pollution in Gary, Indiana 1945–1980* (Chapel Hill and London, 1995).

———, 'Fiasco at Wagner Electric: environmental justice and urban geography in St Louis', *Environmental History*, 4 (1997), 460–81.

Ignatieff, Michael, *A Just Measure of Pain: The Penitentiary in the Industrial Revolution, 1750–1850* (London, 1978).

Illich, Ivan, *Limits to Medicine: Medical Nemesis* (London, 1977).

Inwood, Stephen, *A History of London* (London, 2000).

Jenner, Mark, 'The politics of London air: John Evelyn's *Fumifugium* and the Restoration', *Historical Journal*, 38 (1995), 535–51.

Jones, E.L., *The European Miracle: Environments, Economies and Geopolitics in the History of Europe and Asia* (Cambridge, 1981).

Jones, Greta, *Social Darwinism in English Thought: The Interaction between Biological and Social Theory* (Brighton, 1980).

Jones, Phil, 'The suburban high flat in the post-war reconstruction of Birmingham, 1945–70', *Urban History*, 32 (2005), 308–26.

Kearns, Gerry, 'Aspects of cholera and society and space in nineteenth century England and Wales'. Ph.D. thesis, Cambridge University, 1985.

———, 'Cholera, nuisances and environmental management in Islington, 1830–1855' in W. Bynum and R. Porter (eds), *Living and Dying in London: Medical History Supplement 11* (London, 1991), 94–125.

———, 'Town hall and Whitehall: sanitary intelligence in Liverpool, 1840–63' in Sally Sheard and Helen Power (eds), *Body and City: Histories of Urban Public Health* (Aldershot, 2000), 89–108.

Keith-Lucas, Bryan, *The Unreformed Government System* (London, 1980).

Kellett, J.R., *The Impact of the Railways on Victorian Cities* (London, 1969).

Kermode, Frank, *Shakespeare's Language* (London, 2000).

Kumar, Krishan, 'Versions of the pastoral: poverty and the poor in English fiction from the 1840s to the 1950s', *Journal of Historical Sociology*, 8 (1995), 1–35.

————, *A History of English National Identity* (Cambridge, 2003).

Laberge, A.F., *Mission and Method: The Early Nineteenth Century French Public Health Movement* (Cambridge, 1992).

Lambert, R.S., *Sir John Simon 1816–1904 and English Social Administration* (London,1963).

Lancaster, Brian, 'The "Croydon case": dirty old town to model town: the making of the Croydon Board of Health and the Croydon typhoid epidemic of 1852–3', *Croydon Natural History and Scientific Society*, 18 (2001), 145–206.

Landers, John, *Death and the Metropolis: Studies in the Demographic History of London, 1670–1830* (Cambridge, 1993).

————, 'Urban growth and economic change: from the late seventeenth century to 1841' in Peter Clark (ed.), *Cambridge Urban History of Britain: Volume Two: 1540–1840* (Cambridge, 2000), 453–91.

Laxton, Paul, 'Fighting for public health: Dr Duncan and his adversaries, 1847–63' in Sally Sheard and Helen Power (eds), *Body and City: Histories of Urban Public Health* (Aldershot, 2000), 59–88.

Le Roy Ladurie, E., 'A concept: the unification of the globe by disease (fourteenth to sixteenth centuries)', in Ladurie, *The Mind and Method of the Historian* (Chicago, 1981), 28–83. Translated by S. and B. Reynolds.

Leavis, F.R., *Two Cultures: The Significance of C.P. Snow* (Chatto and Windus, 1962).

Lee, C.H., 'Regional disparities in infant mortality in Britain, 1871–1971: patterns and hypotheses', *Population Studies*, 45 (1991), 55–65.

Lee, Laurie, *Cider with Rosie* (London, 1967).

————, *As I Walked Out One Midsummer Morning* (Harmondsworth, 1971).

Lees, Andrew, *Cities Perceived: Urban Society in European and American Thought 1820–1940* (Manchester, 1985).

Lees, Lynn H., *Exiles of Erin: Irish Migrants in Victorian London* (Manchester, 1979).

————, 'Urban networks' in Martin Daunton (ed.), *Cambridge Urban History: Volume Three:1840–1950* (Cambridge, 2000), 59–94.

LeMahieu, D.L., *A Culture for Democracy: Mass Communication and the Cultivated Mind in Britain between the Wars* (Oxford, 1988).

Lewis, R.A., *Edwin Chadwick and the Public Health Movement 1832–1854* (London, 1952).

Longmate, Norman, *King Cholera* (London, 1966).

Loudon, Irvine. *Death in Childbirth: An International Study of Maternal Care and Maternal Mortality, 1800–1950* (Oxford, 1992).

Lovelock, James, *Gaia: A New Look at Life on Earth* (Oxford, 1979).

Luckin, Bill, *Pollution and Control: A Social History of the Thames in the Nineteenth Century* (Bristol and Boston, 1986).

————, 'Varieties of the environmental', *Journal of Urban History*, 24 (1997–98), 510–23.

————, 'The shaping of a public environmental sphere in late nineteenth century London' in Steve Sturdy (ed.), *Medicine, Health and the Public Sphere in Britain, 1600–2000* (Routledge, 2002), 224–40.

————, 'Revisiting the idea of urban degeneration in Victorian Britain', *Urban History*, 33 (2006), 234–52.

————, 'History, community and utopia: the Manchester reconstruction plan', in Elena Cogato Lanza and Patrizia Bonifazio (eds), *Les Experts de la Reconstruction: Figures et Strategies d'Elite Technique dans L'Europe de L'Apres-Guerre*, (Geneva, 2009), 37–48.

MacLeod, R.M., 'The Alkali Acts administration, 1863–84: the emergence of the civil scientist', *Victorian Studies*, 9 (1965), 85–112.

————, 'Government and resource conservation: the Salmon Acts Administration, 1860–1886', *Journal of British Studies*, 8 (1968), 114–50.

————, 'The X-Club: a social network of science in Victorian England', *Notes and Records of the Royal Society*, 24 (1970), 305–22.

Marks, Lara, *Metropolitan Maternity: Maternal and Infant Welfare Services in Early Twentieth Century London* (Amsterdam and Atlanta, 1996).

Marsh, Jan, *Back to the Land: The Pastoral Impulse in England 1880–1914* (London, 1982).

Marshall, W.A. L., *A Century of London Weather* (London, 1952).

Massard-Guilbaud, Genevieve, *Histoire de la Pollution Industrielle: France 1789–1914* (Paris, 2010).

————, Harold L. Platt and Dieter Schott (eds), *Cities and Catastrophes: Coping with Emergency in European History* (Oxford, 2002).

————, Genevieve and Peter Thorsheim (eds), 'European environmental history', *Journal of Urban History*, 33 (2007), 691–881, special issue.

Matless, David, *Landscape and Englishness* (London, 1998).

McGraw, R.E., *Russia and the Cholera 1823–32* (Madison, 1965).

McKeown, Thomas and R.G. Record, 'Reasons for the decline of mortality in England and Wales during the nineteenth century', *Population Studies*, 16 (1962), 94–122.

————, R.G. Brown and R.G. Record, 'An interpretation of the modern rise of population in Europe', *Population Studies*, 26 (1972), 345–82.

———— *The Modern Rise of Population* (London, 1976).

————, *The Role of Medicine. Dream, Mirage or Nemesis?* (Oxford, 1979).

————, *The Origins of Human Disease* (Oxford, 1988).

McKichan, F., 'A burgh's response to the problems of urban growth: Stirling, 1780–1880', *Scottish Historical Review*, 57 (1978), 68–86.

McNeill, J.R. 'The environment, environmentalism and international society in the long 1970s' in Ferguson, Niall *et al.*, *The Shock of the Global: The 1970s in Perspective* (Cambridge, 2010), 263–78.

McNeill, William H., *Plagues and Peoples* (Oxford, 1977).

Megaw, J.W. D., 'Typhus fevers and other rickettsial fevers' in *The British Encyclopaedia of Medical Practice, Volume 2* (London, 1952).

Mellers, Wilfrid, *Vaughan Williams and the Vision of Albion* (London, 1989).

Melosi, Martin V. (ed.), *Pollution and Reform in American Cities 1870–1930* (Austin, 1980).

————, *Garbage in the City: Refuse, Reform and the Environment 1880–1920* (College Station, 1981).

————, 'The place of the city in environmental history', *Environmental History Review*, 17 (1993), 1–23.

————, 'Equity, eco-racism and environmental history', *Environmental History Review*, 19 (1995), 1–16.

————, *The Sanitary City: Urban Infrastructure in America from Colonial Times to the Present* (Baltimore, 2000).

————, *Effluent America: Cities, Industry, Energy and the Environment* (Pittsburgh, 2001).

Merchant, Carolyn, *The Death of Nature: Women, Ecology and the Scientific Revolution* (London, 1981).

Mitchell, B.R., *International Historical Statistics: Europe 1750–2000* (Basingstoke, 2003).

————. and Phyllis Deane, *Abstract of British Historical Statistics* (Cambridge, 1962).

Monk, Ray, *Bertrand Russell: Volume 1: The Spirit of Solitude* (London, 1996).

Mooney, Graham, Bill Luckin and Andrea Tanner, 'Patient pathways: solving the problem of institutional mortality in the later nineteenth century', *Social History of Medicine*, 12 (1999), 227–69.

————, and Andrea Tanner, 'Infant mortality, a spatial problem: Notting Dale special area' in Eilidh Garrett *et al.*, *Infant Mortality: A Continuing Social Problem* (Aldershot, 2006), 79–98.

————, 'Historical demography and epidemiology: the meta-narrative challenge', in Mark Jackson (ed.), *Oxford Handbook of the History of Medicine* (Oxford, 2011), 373–92.

Moore, James and Richard Rodger, 'Who really ran the cities? Municipal knowledge and policy networks in British local government, 1832–1914', in Ralf Roth and Robert Beachy (eds), *Who Ran the Cities? City Elites and Urban Power Structures in Europe and North America, 1750–1940* (Aldershot, 2007), 37–70.

Morris, R.J., *Cholera 1832: The Social Response to an Epidemic* (London, 1976).

Mosely, Stephen, 'The Manchester and Salford Noxious Vapour Abatement Association, 1876–1895'. M.A. thesis. University of Lancaster, 1994.

————, *The Chimney of the World: A History of Smoke Pollution in Victorian and Edwardian Manchester* (Cambridge, 2001).

————, 'Common ground: integrating social and environmental history', *Journal of Social History*, 39 (2006), 915–33.

Mudhopadhyay, A.K., 'The politics of London water supply, 1871–1971', Ph.D. thesis, University of London. 1972.

Murphy, E.S., 'Typhus fever group' in P.D. Hoeprich (ed.), *Infectious Diseases* (London, 1972), 791–99.

Needham, Joseph and Lu Gwei-Djen, 'Medicine and Chinese culture' in Joseph Needham, *Clerks and Craftsmen in China and the West* (Cambridge, 1970), 263–93.

Newsholme, Arthur, *Fifty Years in Public Health* (London, 1935).

O'Brien, J.V., *'Dear Dirty Dublin': A City in Distress 1899–1916* (Berkeley, 1982).

Obelkevich, James, *Religion and Rural Society: South Lindsey, 1825–1875* (Oxford, 1976).

Oddy, Derek and Derek S. Miller (eds), *The Making of the Modern British Diet* (London, 1976).

Olechnowicz, A., *Working-Class Housing in England between the Wars: The Becontree Estate* (Oxford, 1997).

Ortalano, Guy, *The Two Cultures Controversy: Science, Literature and Politics in Post-war Britain* (Cambridge, 2009).
Owen, David, *The Government of Victorian London, 1855–1889: The Metropolitan Board of Works, the Vestries, and the City Corporation* (Cambridge, 1982), edited by Roy M. MacLeod.
Parry, B., *Conrad and Imperialism: Boundaries and Visionary Fantasies* (London, 1983).
Partington, J.R., *A History of Chemistry, Volume Four* (London, 1964).
Passmore, John, *Man's Responsibility for Nature* (London, 1974).
Patten, R.L., '"A surprising transformation": Dickens and the hearth' in C. Knopflmacher and G.B. Tennyson (eds), *Nature and the Victorian Imagination* (Berkeley, 1977), 153–70.
Pelling, Margaret, 'Some approaches to nineteenth century epidemiology with particular reference to John Snow and William Budd', B. Litt. thesis, University of Oxford. 1971.
———, *Cholera, Fever and English Medicine 1825–1865* (Oxford, 1978).
Pennybacker, S.D., *A Vision for London: London, Everyday Life and the LCC Experiment* (London, 1995).
Perkin, Frank, *Middle-Class Radicalism: The Social Bases of the British Campaign for Nuclear Disarmament* (Manchester, 1968).
Peter, Hennock, 'Urban sanitary reform a generation before Chadwick?', *Economic History Review*, 10 (1957), 113–20.
Pick, Daniel, *Faces of Degenerationism: A European Disorder c. 1848–1914* (Cambridge, 1989).
Picker, John M., 'The sound-proof study: urban professionals, work space and urban noise', *Victorian Studies*, 42 (1999–2000), 427–53.
Platt, Harold L., 'Invisible gases: smoke, gender and the redefinition of environmental policy in Chicago, 1900–1920', *Planning Perspectives*, 10 (1995), 67–97.
———, 'Jane Addams and the ward boss revisited: class, politics and public health in Chicago, 1890–1930', *Environmental History*, 5 (2000), 194–222.
———, *Shock Cities: The Environmental Transformation and Reform of Manchester and Chicago* (Chicago, 2005).
Ponting, Clive, *A Green History of the World* (London, 1992).
Pooley, Colin, 'Patterns on the ground: urban form, residential structure and the social construction of space' in Martin Daunton (ed.), *Cambridge Urban History of Britain: Volume 3: 1840–1950* (Cambridge, 2000), 429–66.
Pooley, M.E. and C.G. Pooley, 'Health, society and environment in nineteenth century Manchester', in Robert Woods and John Woodward (eds), *Urban Disease and Mortality in Nineteenth Century England* (London, 1984), 148–75.
Porter, D.H., *The Thames Embankment: Technology and Society in Victorian London* (Akron, Ohio, 1999).
Porter, Dorothy, '"Enemies of the race": biologism, environmentalism and public health in Edwardian Britain', *Victorian Studies*, 34 (1991), 159–78.
———, and Porter, Roy, *Patient's Progress: Doctors and Doctoring in Eighteenth Century England* (Oxford, 1989).
Porter, Roy and Dorothy Porter, *In Sickness and In Health: The British Experience* (Oxford, 1988).

————, 'Laymen, doctors and medical knowledge in the eighteenth century: the evidence of the *Gentleman's Magazine*' in Roy Porter (ed.), *Patients and Practitioners: Lay Perceptions of Medicine in Pre-Industrial Society* (Cambridge, 1985), 281–314.

————, 'The Patient's View', *Theory and Society*, 14 (1985), 175–98.

————, *Mind-Forg'd Manacles: Madness and Psychiatry in England from the Restoration to the Regency* (Cambridge, 1985).

————, 'Cleaning up in the Great Wen: public health in eighteenth century London' in W.F. Bynum and R.Porter (eds), *Living and Dying in London: Medical History Supplement 11* (London, 1991), 61–75.

Post, J.D., 'Famine, mortality and epidemic disease in the process of modernization', *Economic History Review*, 24 (1976), 14–38.

————, *The Last Great Subsistence Crisis in the Western World* (Baltimore, 1977).

Premble, John, *The Mediterranean Passion: Victorians and Edwardians in the South* (Oxford, 1988).

Priestley, J.B., *English Journey* (London, 1934).

Prochaska, F.K., 'Philanthropy' in F.M.L. Thompson (ed.), *The Cambridge Social History of Britain: Volume 3 1750–1950* (Cambridge, 1990), 357–94.

Ravetz, Alison, *Remaking Cities: Contradictions of the Recent Urban Environment* (London, 1980).

Razzell, Peter., 'An interpretation of the modern rise of population in Europe – a critique', *Population Studies*, 28 (1974), 5–17.

————, *The Conquest of Smallpox: The Impact of Inoculation on Smallpox Mortality in Eighteenth Century Britain* (Firle, 1977).

Redford, A., and I.S. Russell, *The History of Local Government in Manchester, Volume 3: The Last Half Century* (London, 1940).

Reed, Peter, 'Robert Angus Smith and the Alkali Inspectorate' in E. Homburg, Anthony S. Travis and Harm G. Schroter (eds), *The Chemical Industry in Europe 1850–1914* (Dordrecht, 1998), 121–48.

Reeder, David, 'Conclusions: perspectives on metropolitan administrative history' in David Owen, *The Government of Victorian London 1855–1889: The Metropolitan Board of Works, the Vestries and the City Corporation*, edited by Roy Macleod. (Cambridge, 1982), 347–69.

Rees, R., 'The South Wales copper-smoke dispute, 1828–95', *Welsh History Review*, 10 (1981), 480–96.

Reid Donald, *Paris Sewers and Sewermen: Realities and Representations* (Cambridge, 1991).

Richmond, P., *Marketing Modernisms; The Architecture and Influence of Charles Reilly* (Liverpool, 2001).

Riley, James C., *Sick Not Dead: The Health of British Workingmen during the Mortality Decline* (Baltimore, 1998).

Roberts, Glynn, *Aspects of Welsh History* (Cardiff, 1969).

Roberts, Robert, *The Classic Slum: Salford Life in the First Quarter of the Century* (Manchester, 1971).

Robinson, Alan, *Imagining London, 1770–1900* (London, 2005).

Robson, W.A, *The Government and Misgovernment of London* (London, 1939).

Rodger, Richard, *Edinburgh and the Transformation of the Nineteenth Century City: Land, Property and Trust* (New York and Oxford, 2000).

Rootes, Christopher, 'Environmental protest in Britain, 1988–1997', in B. Seel, M. Paterson and B. Doherty (eds), *Direct Action in British Environmental Protest* (London, 2000), 25–61.

———, *Environmental Protest in Western Europe* (Oxford, 2003).

Rosen, C.M. and J.A. Tarr, 'The importance of an urban perspective in environmental history', *Journal of Urban History*, 20 (1994), 299–310.

Rosen, G., 'Disease, debility and death', in H.J. Dyos and Michael Wolff (eds), *The Victorian City: Images and Realities: Volume 2* (London, 1973), 625–67.

Rosenberg, Charles, *The Cholera Years: The United States in 1832, 1849 and 1866* (Chicago, 1962).

Rosenthal, Michael, *British Landscape Painting* (Oxford, 1982).

Roth, Ralf and Robert Beachy (eds), *Who Ran the Cities? City Elites and Urban Power Structures in Europe and North America, 1750–1940* (Aldershot, 2007).

Russell, Bertrand and Patricia Russell (eds), *The Amberley Papers: Bertrand Russell's Family Background: Volume 2* (London, 1937).

Russell, Colin A., *Edward Frankland: Chemistry, Controversy and Conspiracy in Victorian England* (Cambridge, 1996).

Said, Edward, *Culture and Imperialism* (London, 1978).

Saint, Andrew, (ed.), *Politics and the People of London: The London County Council 1889–1965* (London, 1989).

Saul, S.B., *The Myth of the Great Depression* (London, 1969).

Schneider, Daniel, *Hybrid Nature: Sewage Treatment and the Contradictions of the Industrial Ecosystem* (Cambridge, 2011).

Schoenwald, R.L., 'Training urban man', in H.J. Dyos and Michael Wolff (eds), *The Victorian City: Images and Realities* (London, 1978), 669–92.

Schott, Dieter (ed.), *Energy and the City in Europe: From Preindustrial Wood Shortage to the Oil Crisis of the 1970s* (Stuttgart, 1997).

———, 'Resources of the City: Towards a European Urban Environmental History' in Dieter Schott, Bill Luckin and Genevieve Massard-Guilbaud (eds), *Resources of the City: Contributions to an Environmental History of Modern Europe* (Aldershot, 2005), 1–27.

Schwarz, L.D., *London in the Age of Industrialization: Entrepreneurs, Labour Force and Living Conditions, 1700–1850* (Cambridge, 1992).

———, 'London 1700–1840' in P. Clark (ed.), *Cambridge Urban History of Britain: Volume 2: 1540–1840* (Cambridge, 2000), 641–72.

Schweber, Libby, *Disciplining Statistics: Demography and Vital Statistics in France and England, 1830–1885* (London, 2006).

Scull, Andrew, *Museums of Madness: The Social Origins of Insanity in Nineteenth-Century England* (London, 1979).

Searle, G.R., *Eugenics and Politics in Britain 1900–1914* (Leyden, 1976).

———, *A New England: Peace and War 1886–1914* (Oxford, 2004).

Sharpe, Pamela, 'Population and society 1700–1840' in P. Clark (ed.), *Cambridge Urban History: Volume 2: 1540–1840* (Cambridge, 2000), 491–528.

Sheail, John, 'Public interest and self-interest: the disposal of trade effluent in inter-war Britain', *Twentieth Century British History*, 4 (1993), 149–70.

———, 'Sewering the English suburbs: an inter-war perspective', *Journal of Historical Geography*, 19 (1993), 433–47.

————, '"Taken for granted": the inter-war West Middlesex Drainage Scheme', *London Journal*, 18 (1993), 143–56.

————, 'Town wastes, agricultural sustainability and Victorian sewage', *Urban History*, 23 (1996), 189–210.

————, *An Environmental History of Twentieth Century Britain* (Basingstoke, 2002).

Sheppard, Francis W., *London 1808–1870: The Infernal Wen* (London, 1971).

————, *London: A History* (Oxford, 1998).

Shortland, Michael (ed.), *Science and Nature* (Stamford-in-the-Vale, 1993).

————, 'Cholera in the large towns of the West and East Ridings, 1843–1983', Ph. D. thesis, Sheffield University, 1991.

————, and Michael Worboys, 'The public's view of public health in mid-Victorian Britain', *Urban History*, 21 (1994), 237–50.

Simmons, I.G., *An Environmental History of Britain: From 10,000 Years Ago to the Present* (Edinburgh, 2001).

Simo, Louise Melanie, *Loudon and Landscape: From Country Seat to Metropolis 1783–1843* (New Haven, 1988).

Simon, E.D., *How to Abolish the Slums* (London, 1929).

————, *The Anti-Slum Campaign* (London, 1933).

————, *The Rebuilding of Britain: A Twenty Year Plan* (London, 1942).

Singer, Charles and E.A. Underwood, *A Short History of Medicine* (Oxford, 1962).

Smith, D.F., H.L. Diack and T.H. Pennington, *Food Poisoning, Policy and Politics: Corned Beef and Typhoid in Britain in the 1960s* (Woodbridge, 2005).

Smith, F.B., *The People's Health 1830–1910* (London, 1979).

————, *The Retreat of Tuberculosis 1850–1950* (London, 1988).

Smith, P.J., 'The foul burns of Edinburgh: public health attitudes and environmental change', *Scottish Geographical Magazine*, 91 (1975), 25–37.

————, 'The legislated control over river pollution in Victorian Scotland', *Scottish Geographical Magazine*, 98 (1982), 66–76.

Smout, T.C., *Nature Contested: Environmental History in Scotland and North England since 1600* (Edinburgh, 2000).

Snow, C.P., *The Two Cultures and the Scientific Revolution* (New York, 1959).

Snyder, J.C., 'The typhus fevers' in T.M. Rivers (ed.), *Viral and Rickettsial Infections of Man* (Philadelphia, 1952), 578–610.

Spengler, Oswald, *The Decline of the West* (New York, 1966).

Stapleton, Julia, *Sir Arthur Bryant and National History in Twentieth-century Britain* (Lanham, 2005).

Stedman Jones, Gareth, *Outcast London: A Study in the Relationship between Classes in Victorian Society* (Oxford, 1971).

Steere-Williams, Jacob, 'The perfect food and the filth disease: milk, typhoid fever and the science of state medicine in Victorian Britain, 1850–1900'. Ph.D. thesis, University of Minnesota, 2011.

————, 'The perfect food and the filth disease: milk-borne typhoid and epidemiological practice in late Victorian Britain', *Journal of the History of Medicine and Allied Sciences*, 65 (2010), 514–45.

Stevenson, John, and Chris Cook, *The Slump: Society and Politics during the Depression* (London, 1977).

————, *British Society 1914–45* (Harmondsworth, 1984).

Stewart, F.S., *Bigger's Handbook of Bacteriology* (London, 1962).

Stone, Dan, *Breeding Supermen: Nietzsche, Race and Eugenics in Interwar Britain*, (Liverpool, 2002).

Stone, Lawrence, *The Crisis of the Aristocracy* (Oxford, 1965).

Stradling, David, and Peter Thorsheim, 'The smoke of great cities: British and American efforts to control air pollution', *Environmental History*, 4 (1999), 6–31.

——, *Smokestacks and Progressives: Environmentalists, Engineers, and Air Quality 1881–1951* (Baltimore, 1999).

Sunderland, David, 'A monument to defective administration? The London Commission of Sewers in the early nineteenth century', *Urban History*, 26 (1999), 349–372.

Synder, John C., 'The typhus fevers', in Thomas M. Rivers (ed.), *Viral and Rickettsial Infections of Man* (Philadelphia, 1952), 578–610.

Szasz, A., *Ecopoulism: Toxic Waste and the Movement for Environmental Justice* (Minneapolis, 1994).

Szreter, Simon, 'The GRO and the public health movement in Britain, 1837–1914', *Social History of Medicine*, 3 (1991), 435–62.

——, 'Economic growth, disruption, deprivation and death: on the importance of the politics of public health for development' in Szreter, *Health and Wealth: Studies in History and Policy* (Rochester, 2005), 203–41.

—— and Graham Mooney, 'Urbanization, mortality and the standard of living debate: new estimates of the expectation of life in nineteenth-century British cities', *The Economic History Review*, 1 (1998), 84–112.

——, and Anne Hardy, 'Urban fertility and mortality patterns' in Martin Daunton (ed.), *The Cambridge Urban History of Britain: Volume 3: 1750–1840* (Cambridge, 2000), 629–72.

Tarr, Joel A., *The Search for the Ultimate Sink: Urban Pollution in Historical Perspective* (Akron, Ohio, 1995).

——, 'The metabolism of the industrial city: the case of Pittsburgh', *Journal of Urban History*, 28 (2002), 511–45.

Thomas, Brinley, *Migration and Economic Growth: Great Britain and the Atlantic Economy* (Cambridge, 1954).

Thomas, Keith, *Religion and the Decline of Magic: Studies in Popular Beliefs in Sixteenth and Seventeenth Century England* (London, 1971).

——, *Man and the Natural World: Changing Attitudes in England 1500–1800* (New York, 1983).

Thompson, Barbara, 'Infant mortality in nineteenth-century Bradford' in Robert Woods and John Woodward (eds), *Urban Disease and Mortality in Nineteenth-Century England* (London, 1984), 120–47.

Thompson, E.P., *The Making of the English Working Class* (London, 1963).

Thompson, F.M.L., *Hampstead: Building a Borough, 1650–1954* (London, 1974).

——, (ed.), *The Rise of Suburbia* (Leicester, 1982).

——, 'Town and city' in F.M.L. Thompson (ed.), *The Cambridge Social History of Britain. Volume 1: 1750–1850* (Cambridge, 1990), 1–86.

Thompson, John B., *Ideology and Modern Culture: Critical Social Theory in the Era of Mass Communication* (Cambridge, 1990).

Thorsheim, Peter, 'Interpreting the London fog disaster of 1952' in E. Melanie Dupuis (ed.), *Smoke and Mirrors: The Politics and Culture of Air Pollution* (New York, 2004), 154–69.

————, *Inventing Pollution: Coal Smoke and Culture in Britain since 1800* (Athens, Ohio, 2006).

Tinker, H.S., 'The problem', in Institution of Civil Engineers, *Advances in Sewage Treatment* (London, 1973).

Tomes, Nancy, *The Gospel of Germs: Men, Women and the Microbe in American Life* (Cambridge, 1998).

Townsend, P., N. Davidson and M. Whitehead (eds), *Inequalities in Health: The Black Report* (Harmondsworth, 1988).

Trainor, R.H., *Authority and Social Structure in an Industrial Area: A Study of Three Black Country Towns* (Oxford, 1981).

Trevelyan, G.M., *Must England's Beauty Perish? A Plea on Behalf of the National Trust for Places of Historic Interest and Natural Beauty* (London, 1929).

————, *English Social History; a Survey of Six Centuries, Chaucer to Queen Victoria* (London, 1942).

Ulrich Beck. *The Risk Society: Towards a New Modernity*, translated by M. Rimmer. (London, 1992).

Vannatta, D.P., H.E. Bates (Boston, 1983).

Vernon, Jenson, J., 'The X-Club: a fraternity of Victorian scientists', *British Journal for the History of Science*, 5 (1970–1), 63–72.

Vinten-Johansen, Peter et al., *Cholera, Chloroform and the Science of Medicine* (Oxford, 2003).

von Tunzelmann, G.N., 'Trends in real wages, 1750–1850, revisited', *Economic History Review*, 32 (1979), 33–49.

Walkowitz, Judith, *City of Dreadful Delight: Narratives of Sexual Danger in Late Victorian Britain* (Chicago, 1992).

Waller, P.J., *Town, City and Nation* (Oxford, 1983).

Weaver, Stewart A., *The Hammonds: A Marriage in History* (Stanford, 1997).

Weber, Gay, 'Science and society in nineteenth century anthropology', *History of Science*, 7 (1974), 260–83.

Welsh, Ian, *Mobilising Modernity: The Nuclear Movement* (London, 2000).

Wheeler, A., *The Tidal Thames* (London, 1979).

White, Jerry, *London in the Twentieth Century: A City and its People* (London, 2001).

Wilkinson, Richard, *Unhealthy Societies: The Afflictions of Inequality* (London, 1996).

Williams-Ellis, Clough, *England and the Octopus* (London, 1928).

————, (ed.), *Britain and the Beast* (London, 1937).

Williams, Naomi, 'Death in its season: class, environment and the mortality of infants in nineteenth century Britain', *Social History of Medicine*, 5 (1992), 71–94.

————, and Graham Mooney, 'Infant mortality in an "age of great cities": London and the English provincial cities compared, c. 1840–1910', *Continuity and Change*, 9 (1994), 185–212.

————, and Chris Galley, 'Urban-rural differentials in infant mortality in Victorian England', *Population Studies*, 49 (1995), 401–20.

Williams, Raymond, *The Country and the City* (London, 1973).

Williams, Rosalind, *Notes on the Underground: An Essay on Technology, Society and the Imagination* (Cambridge, 1990).

Williamson, J.G., *Coping with City Growth during the British Industrial Revolution* (Cambridge, 1990).

————, 'Did England's cities grow too fast during the Industrial Revolution?' in P. Higonnet, D.S. Landes and H. Rosovsky (eds), *Favorites of Fortune: Technology, Growth and Economic Development since the Industrial Revolution* (Cambridge, 1991), 359–94.

Williamson, Philip, *Stanley Baldwin: Conservative Leadership and National Values* (Cambridge, 1999).

Wilson, A., 'Technology and municipal decision-making: sanitary systems in Manchester, 1868–1910', Ph.D. thesis, University of Manchester, 1990.

Winner, Langdon, 'Upon opening the black box and finding it empty: social constructivism and the philosophy of technology', *Science, Technology and Human Values*, 18 (1993), 362–78.

Winter, J.M., *Sites of Memory, Sites of Mourning: The Great War in English Cultural History* (Cambridge, 1995).

Winter, James, *London's Teeming Streets 1830–1914* (London, 1993).

————, *Secure from Rash Assault: Sustaining the Victorian Environment* (Berkeley, 1999).

Wohl, A.S., 'The housing of the working classes in London, 1815–1914' in S.D. Chapman (ed.), *The History of Working-Class Housing: A Symposium* (Newton Abbott, 1971), 15–54.

————, 'Unfit for human habitation' in H.J. Dyos and M. Wolff (eds), *The Victorian City: Images and Realities: Volume One* (London, 1973), 603–24.

————, *The Eternal Slum: Housing and Social Policy in Victorian London* (London, 1977).

————, *Endangered Lives: Public Health in Victorian Britain* (London, 1983).

Wood, L.B., *The Restoration of the Tidal Thames* (Bristol, 1982).

Woods, Robert, 'Mortality and sanitary conditions in the "best governed city in the world" – Birmingham, 1870–1910', *Journal of Historical Geography*, 4 (1978), 35–56.

———— and John Woodward (eds), *Urban Disease and Mortality in Nineteenth Century England* (London, 1984).

————, and Nicola Shelton, *An Atlas of Victorian Mortality* (Liverpool, 1997).

————, *The Demography of Victorian England and Wales* (Cambridge, 2000).

Worboys, Michael, *Spreading Germs: Disease Theories and Medical Practice in Britain 1865–1900* (Cambridge, 2000).

Worster, Donald, 'Transformations of the earth: towards an agroecological perspective in history', *Journal of American History*, 76 (1989), 1087–100.

Wright, A., *Foreign Country: The Life of L.P. Hartley* (London, 1996).

Wrigley, E.A., 'A simple model of London's importance in changing English society and economy 1650–1750', *Past and Present*, 37 (1967), 44–70.

Wynne, Brian, *Rationality and Ritual: The Windscale Inquiry and Nuclear Decisions in Britain* (Chalfont St Giles, 1982).

Young, Ken and Patricia L. Garside, *Metropolitan London: Politics and Urban Change, 1837–1981* (London, 1982).

Zinsser, Hans., 'Varieties of typhus virus and the epidemiology of the American form of European typhus fever (Brill's disease)', *American Journal of Hygiene* 20 (1934), 513–32.

————, *Rats, Lice and History* (London, 1935).

INDEX

history, London County Council,
typhoid, typhus, urban provincial
Britain, water supply
London County Council, 12, 52,
69–72, 85–8. *See also* London,
Metropolitan Board of Works
London Fever Hospital, 39, 40, 41
London Hospital Cholera Fund, 10
Louis, P.C.A., 38

MacLeod, Roy, 111
Makins, W.T., 127
Manchester, 11, 73, 80, 81, 144, 151,
170, 173, 183
Manchester and Salford Noxious Vapours
Abatement Association, 112
Mansion House Cholera Relief Fund, 10
Marylebone, 42
McKeown, Thomas, 4, 6, 46, 50, 144
McNamara, T.J., 86
Medical Office of the Privy Council, 78
Melosi, Martin, 119, 159
Merthyr Tydfil, 171
Metropolitan Asylums Board, 8, 53, 69,
70
Metropolitan Board of Works, 12, 53,
69, 76, 80, 81
Metropolitan Commission of Sewers, 84
Metropolitan Water Act, 1852, 58
Metropolitan Water Board, 76, 88
Miasmatic theory, 15
Midleton, Viscount, 128
Migration, 145
Morbidity and mortality, 10, 8–9,
26–7, 193n.33 *See also* Disease
Morris, William, 145
Municipal Corporations Act 1835, 82,
83
Murphy, Shirley Forster, 52–3, 72, 77

Nash, Paul, 143
National Audubon Society, 157
National Smoke Abatement
Institution, 126

National Trust, 164
National Wildlife Federation, 157
Needham, Joseph, 23
Newcastle, 183, 184
New River Company, 47, 52
Norwich, 73, 170, 183
Notting Dale, London, 72
Nottingham, 171

Orton, Thomas, 60–1, 66–7
Oxford, 186
Owen, David, 75

Palmerston, Lord, 97
Pasteur, Louis, 61
Pelling, Margaret, 174
Pollution problems, conceptualization,
17, 93–5; conflict between
town and country, 95, 98–9;
legislative control, 96–7;
'quasi-solutions', 98–9; small
town experiences, 14; social
construction, 93; spatial and
industrial triggers, 94;
transposition, 95. *See also* Great
London Fogs, London, river pollution, smoke, smoke problems
Platt, Harold, 156, 161
Porter, R.S., 118
Port of London Authority, 69, 88
Preston, 171
Public Health Act 1875, 108

Radcliffe, John Netten, 9, 10, 65–6,
67, 68
'Random' ecological change, 31
Record, R.G., 53
Redford, Arthur, 100
Reeder, David, 69
Regional variations in health, 72–4,
183–5
Regulating the sick poor, 181
Reports of the Registrar-General, 25
River Lea Trust, 59